Case Studies in Medical Toxicology

Leslie R. Dye • Christine Murphy
Diane P. Calello • Michael D. Levine
Aaron Skolnik
Editors

Case Studies in Medical Toxicology

From the American College of Medical Toxicology

Medical Toxicology Foundation

Springer

ACMT | American College of Medical Toxicology

Editors
Leslie R. Dye
Editor-in-Chief, Point of Care Content
Elsevier Clinical Solutions
Cincinnati, OH, USA

Diane P. Calello
Division of Medical Toxicology
Department of Emergency Medicine
Rutgers New Jersey Medical School
Newark, NJ, USA

Aaron Skolnik
Department of Critical Care Medicine
University of Pittsburgh Medical Center
Pittsburgh, PA, USA

Christine Murphy
Department of Emergency Medicine
Divisions of Medical Toxicology and
Pediatric Emergency Medicine
Carolinas Medical Center
Charlotte, NC, USA

Michael D. Levine
Department of Emergency Medicine
Division of Medical Toxicology
University of Southern California
Los Angeles, CA, USA

ISBN 978-3-319-56447-0 ISBN 978-3-319-56449-4 (eBook)
DOI 10.1007/978-3-319-56449-4

Library of Congress Control Number: 2017948728

Printed on acid-free paper

This Springer imprint is published by Springer Nature
The registered company is Springer International Publishing AG
The registered company address is: Gewerbestrasse 11, 6330 Cham, Switzerland

LD: For my husband, Brian, and my parents, Bernice and Ray—a perfect combination.

CM: Geoff, without your tolerance of the chaos around me, none of this would be possible. You are my rock.

DC: To my family, without whom nothing would be possible.

ML: This book is dedicated to my wife Ilene Claudius, and my parents Carol and Murray Levine.

AS: To the loves of my life, Jessica and Asher Lev.

Foreword

Medical toxicology, a specialty of medicine focused on the prevention, diagnosis, and management of human poisoning, is a discipline of stories. Unlike most illness, in which a disease insidiously overtakes a patient, poisoning is often a discrete, definable event. Viewed as a spectator, the event would appear as an unfolding series of foreseeable actions leading to an unintended culmination: poisoning. The child left alone with the bathroom cabinet ajar, the worker reaching for the "water bottle," the depressed patient attempting to end their anguish, the injection drug user buying from a new supplier, each representing a common scenario in which poisoning occurs. What happens next depends on many variables such as the nature, dose, and route of exposure, the size, age, and health of the patient, the set and setting, the recognition of the event, and even the availability and timely administration of the specific antidote.

Considering the many permutations, each of these unfolding stories requires skill to piece together in a logical and orderly manner. Prognosis guides expectation, and treatment quells fear. The knowledge and experience to understand the natural history of various poisonings are part of the early training necessary to become a medical toxicologist. This is a specialty of Sherlock Holmes-like detective work, in which no clues can be left untouched. Just as a single carbon separates an evening of gregarious enjoyment (ethanol) from a lifetime of blindness (methanol), no detail can be considered too small.

For several years, the American College of Medical Toxicology (ACMT), the professional organization of medical toxicologists, has held a monthly member-only, case-based webinar. During this time, I have led hundreds of participants on a journey to dissect complicated, intriguing human poisonings, while each shared their thoughts and beliefs on the how's and why's of medical management. Each case was initially selected for presentation because it was a challenge to someone, and on this basis it served as a learning tool for medical toxicologists across the USA and, often, across the world.

In this book, a group of dedicated medical toxicologists and gifted clinician educators have faithfully reproduced the case discussions, added detail, filled in blanks, and corrected errors, to allow others who were not able to engage in the initial process to benefit from the work of the participants. The cases are anonymized, but nonetheless represent the potential for real life exposures that can, in an instant or over a decade, lead to consequential adverse effects on human health. To increase the value of the book, each case is followed by a discussion of key issues to broaden out the relevance to other medical specialties.

I want to thank the editors (Christina, Diane, Aaron, and Michael) for their tireless attention to detail. A particularly special thanks goes to the champion of the process, Leslie, for making this labor of love a reality. Hopefully their combined efforts will inspire the readers of the book to savor the intriguing tales, while reminding each of us about our tenuous relationship with the chemical milieu in which we live.

Division of Medical Toxicology,
Department of Emergency Medicine
Rutgers New Jersey Medical School,
Newark, NJ, USA

Lewis S. Nelson

Preface

In 2011, the American College of Medical toxicology began offering webinars to members entitled, "National Case Conference." Real medical toxicology cases were presented by people from various training programs and were moderated by seasoned medical toxicologists. The popularity and educational value were quickly recognized and the webinars continue every month. The cases are usually presented by medical toxicology fellows, but sometimes also presented by residents or medical toxicologists who are faculty members. Listeners participate by asking and answering questions.

The format used produced valuable information that the editors thought would be an excellent foundation for a book of cases. Five prominent medical toxicologists, the lead editor an immediate past president of the American College of Medical Toxicology, edited all of the included cases. In addition, the editors added questions and answers that cover various aspects of medical toxicology, to allow readers to test their knowledge on a variety of toxicology topics. At the end of each case, specialty-specific guidance was added to broaden the appeal to providers in primary care and intensive care. This volume is a necessary resource for medical students, residents, and fellows, as well as seasoned medical providers.

Cincinnati, OH	Leslie R. Dye
Charlotte, NC	Christine Murphy
Newark, NJ	Diane P. Calello
Los Angeles, CA	Michael D. Levine
Pittsburgh, PA	Aaron Skolnik

Acknowledgements

The editors would like to acknowledge the American College of Medical Toxicology, the organizers of the National Case Conference, and, most importantly, all of the patients and healthcare workers involved in these cases.

Disclaimer: NCC is an educational endeavor and a quality improvement effort intended to improve patient care. The cases in this book are not intended to define standard of care. Attempts have been made to ensure HIPAA compliance.

All data and information provided in this activity is for informational purposes only. The American College of Medical Toxicology and the editors and contributors of this book make no representations as to accuracy, completeness, present acceptability, suitability, or validity of the content and will not be liable for any errors or omissions in this information or any losses, injuries, or damages arising from its display or use.

Contents

About the Editors

Leslie R. Dye, M.D., F.A.C.M.T. graduated from the University of Kansas School of Medicine and completed a residency in Emergency Medicine and fellowship in Medical Toxicology and Hyperbaric Medicine at the University of Cincinnati. She served as the Editor-in-Chief of the *Journal of Medical Toxicology*, has authored numerous book chapters, and has published extensively in the scientific literature. She currently serves as the Editor-in-Chief of Point of Care Content for Elsevier in addition to practicing addiction medicine. Dr. Dye is board certified in Emergency Medicine and Medical Toxicology and is the immediate past president of the American College of Medical Toxicology and the past president of the Medical Toxicology Foundation.

Christine Murphy, M.D. received both her bachelor's and master's degrees in chemistry from the College of William and Mary and her medical degree from the Medical College of Virginia. She completed her residency training in Emergency Medicine at Virginia Commonwealth University and a fellowship in Medical Toxicology at Carolinas Medical Center. She is currently an Assistant Professor at Carolinas Medical Center and Director of the Medical Toxicology Fellowship Program. Dr. Murphy is board certified in Emergency Medicine and Medical Toxicology. Her current interests include alternative uses for existing antidotes and trends in recreational drugs of abuse.

Diane P. Calello, M.D., F.A.C.M.T. is the Executive and Medical Director of the New Jersey Poison Information and Education System at the New Jersey Medical School of Rutgers University. She is also a member of the Board of Directors of the American College of Medical Toxicology and a regular contributor to the National Case Conference Webinar.She received her Bachelor of Arts from the College of William and Mary in Virginia and her medical degree from the New Jersey Medical School she now calls home. Her residency and fellowship training was conducted at the Children's Hospital of Philadelphia.She is board certified in Pediatrics, Pediatric Emergency Medicine,

Medical Toxicology, and Addiction Medicine. Dr. Calello is a national expert on pediatric lead poisoning, use of critical care methods in poisoning patients, and the impact of the opioid and emerging drug epidemic on the young child.

Michael D. Levine, M.D., F.A.C.M.T. After matriculating from the Chicago Medical School, Dr. Michael Levine completed an emergency medicine residency at the Brigham and Women's/Massachusetts General Hospital. He subsequently attended the Banner Good Samaritan Medical Center in Phoenix, Arizona, where he completed his medical toxicology fellowship. Michael Levine is currently faculty at the University of Southern California, where he serves as Chief of the Division of Medical Toxicology. His current research interests are mostly focused on toxicity from antiplatelets and anticoagulants. He is on the editorial board of the *Journal of Medical Toxicology*.

Aaron Skolnik, M.D. received his Medical Doctorate from the University of Pittsburgh School of Medicine and completed residency in emergency medicine at Brigham and Women's/Massachusetts General Hospital in Boston, MA. Thereafter, Aaron graduated from the medical toxicology fellowship at Banner Good Samaritan Medical Center in Phoenix, AZ, and joined the faculty of the University of Arizona College of Medicine, Phoenix. He is board certified in Emergency Medicine, Medical Toxicology, and Addiction Medicine. Currently, he is completing additional fellowship training at the University of Pittsburgh in critical care medicine, neurocritical care, and extracorporeal life support.

Case 1
Laundry Pod Ingestion in an Adult

1. Should we be concerned about laundry detergent (LD) pod exposures?
2. How are LD pods different from traditional LD products?
3. How should patients with LD pod exposures be managed?
4. What is being done to reduce harm from LD pod exposures?

Abstract Laundry detergent (LD) pod ingestion is an increasing source of morbidity and mortality in the pediatric population. However, injury associated with unintentional ingestions of LD pods by adults has not been described in the literature. We report a case of a 50-year-old man who ingested a LD pod and had esophageal and gastric injuries.

Keywords Laundry • Detergent • Pod • Caustics • Aspiration

Emergency Department Presentation

Chief Complaint: 50-year-old man presents with vomiting and odynophagia.

History of Present Illness

A 50-year-old hypertensive man who could not read English drank the contents of a Tide Pods® laundry detergent (LD) pod, mistaking it for candy. He vomited immediately after the ingestion and developed repeated emesis over the next 6 h. His

L.R. Dye et al. (eds.), *Case Studies in Medical Toxicology*,
DOI 10.1007/978-3-319-56449-4_1

efforts to eat and drink caused pain and repeated vomiting. The patient presented to ED 12 h after the ingestion, complaining of odynophagia.

Past Medical History	Hypertension
Medications	None
Allergies	None
Social History	Denied drinking alcohol, smoking cigarettes, and using illicit drugs

Physical Examination

Blood pressure	Heart rate	Respiratory rate	Temperature	O_2 saturation
185/111 mmHg	83 bpm	16 breaths/min	36.4 °C (97.6 °F)	97%

General: Lying in a gurney, comfortable
HEENT: Normocephalic with normal pupils, normal tongue, and oropharynx; no evidence of oropharyngeal burns
Cardiovascular: Regular rate and rhythm with no murmurs
Pulmonary: Symmetric breath sounds; lungs were clear to auscultation with no rales or rhonchi
Abdominal: Normal bowel sounds, soft, non-distended, and non-tender
Neurologic: Alert and oriented to person, place, and time; answered all questions appropriately
Skin: Warm and well-perfused

Diagnostic Testing

WBC	Hemoglobin	Hematocrit	Platelets
9.2 K/μL	15.2 g/dL	45%	223 K/dL

Na	K	Cl	CO_2	BUN	Cr	Glucose
139 mEq/L	4.0 mEq/L	103 mEq/L	27 mEq/L	16 mg/dL	0.8 mg/dL	98 mg/dL

Ancillary Testing

An esophagogastroduodenoscopy (EGD) performed in the ED revealed diffuse superficial erythema and ulcerations to the esophagus (Zargar's grade 2A) and stomach (Fig. A–D).

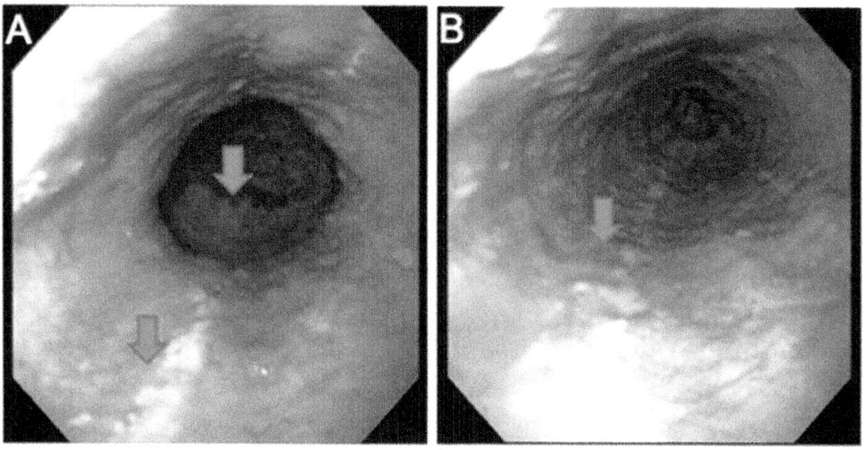

Fig. A, B Grade 2A esophageal injuries

Fig. C Antral and pyloric ulcers

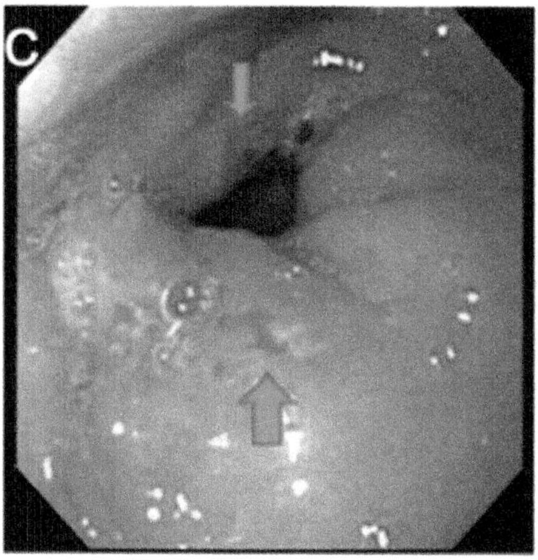

Fig. D Gastric mucosal erythema

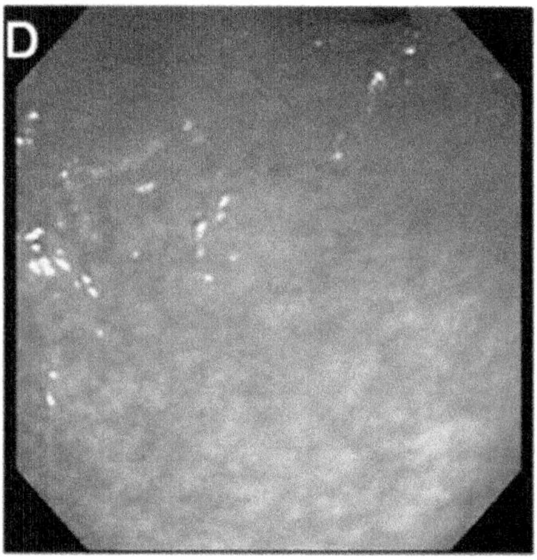

Treatment and Hospital Course

The patient was managed with a proton pump inhibitor and given a liquid diet overnight. He had no further episodes of vomiting while in the hospital, and his odynophagia resolved. He was discharged the following day.

Key Points of Case

Should We Be Concerned About LD Pod Exposures?

In 2012, single-dose LD capsules emerged in the US market as a new, more convenient replacement for the liquid form. These colorful, attractive capsules can resemble candy or toys, likely playing an important role in the alarming number of pediatric exposures. From 2012 through 2103, poison control centers (PCC) in the US received over 17,000 calls reporting LD pod exposures in the pediatric population (Valdez et al. 2014). This astounding number represents less than 2 years of data collection and is likely an underrepresentation of the true exposure.

From 2012 through 2013, LD pod exposures required higher levels of care than pediatric exposures overall. (Valdez et al. 2014). Exposures in adults are much more uncommon. Pod exposures resulted in more than five times the serious outcomes compared to the traditional liquids and powders (Forrester 2013). A study looking into data from PCC recorded 102 children requiring tracheal intubation and two pediatric deaths associated with LD pod exposures (Valdez et al. 2014).

How Are LD Pods Different from Traditional Laundry Products?

Typically, unintentional ingestions of traditional detergent powders and liquids result in minimal toxicity; primarily gastrointestinal effects of mild mouth irritation and transient vomiting (Fulton 2011). The newer LD pod formulation has been available in Europe for a decade and has been associated with more significant morbidity. Although there are differences based on manufacturers, LD pods usually contain primarily ethoxylated alcohols, propylene glycol, and linear alkylbenzene sulfonate enclosed within a water-soluble polyvinyl alcohol membrane (Buehler et al. 2013).

LD pod ingestions result in many of the same gastrointestinal findings as their non-pod counterparts. However, pod ingestions appear to be associated with a greater degree of drowsiness/lethargy, coma, and loss of airway than ingestion of non-pod detergent formulations (Buehler et al. 2013; Forrester 2013). It is unclear if these central effects are due to the ethoxylated alcohol or propylene glycol component, or both. It also remains unclear if exposed adults would share these similar neurologic findings.

How Should Patients with LD Pod Exposures Be Managed?

The initial management of LD pod ingestions is primarily supportive care.

Patients may or may not exhibit oropharyngeal irritation and burns, but as with other caustic exposures, these findings (or lack of) are not reliable predictors of esophageal and gastric injuries. Since there is no reliable relationship between oropharyngeal injuries and esophageal injuries, Crain et al. suggest that patients with a caustic exposure and two or more serious symptoms (vomiting, drooling, and stridor) should undergo endoscopy (Crain et al. 1984).

Studies looking specifically at esophageal injuries after LD pod ingestions are limited. The few case series and reports have found only superficial injury and none have reported any cases of esophageal strictures (Smith et al. 2014; Bramuzzo et al. 2013; Williams et al. 2012). Although the viscosity of the LD pod ingredients should limit its ability to cause distal injury, the ease of consuming larger quantities and the mode of delivery make injury difficult to predict. The decision to perform an EGD on patients who have ingested LD pods should depend on their presentation and progress.

What Is Being Done to Reduce Harm from LD Pod Exposures?

In May 2012, the American Association of Poison Control Centers sounded a nationwide alarm by issuing a release detailing safety precautions. Procter & Gamble (P&G), the maker of Tide Pods® LD pods, and other manufacturers responded with educational campaigns, appended warnings to its advertisements, and placed stickers on the container tubs to remind users to keep the products away from children. P&G has added latches to the lid of their product containers to make them harder to open (Ng 2013). They have also replaced the clear containers with opaque ones to decrease visibility to children.

The most recent data suggest that LD pod exposures may be on the decline; however, it is not yet clear if the decline is a result of harm reduction strategies or a seasonal trend in the number of PCC calls reporting exposures (Valdez et al. 2014). It is unknown whether the pod containers of any brand are truly child-resistant, and currently, there are no standards for safe packaging. Further research is needed to determine which components of the LD pods are most toxic. Once the most dangerous ingredients are determined, product reformulation may mitigate harm.

Specialty-Specific Guidance

Emergency Medicine

- Exposure to LD pods results in more severe adverse effects than exposure to traditional LD powders/liquids.
- Symptoms associated with LD pod include:
  - Gastrointestinal

    Vomiting
    Nausea
    Oropharyngeal irritation
    Abdominal pain
    Diarrhea
  - Neurologic

    Drowsiness
    Lethargy
    Agitation/irritability
    Coma
  - Pulmonary

    Coughing/choking
    Dyspnea
    Respiratory depression
    Pneumonitis
- Management
  - Management for LD pod ingestions is largely supportive
  - EGD according to clinical picture
  - Tracheal intubation when needed

Public Health

- Exposure to LD pods requires more medical attention, hospitalizations, and intensive care than exposures to traditional LD products.
- Public health efforts have resulted in a recent decrease in LD pod exposures, but safety standards still need to be established.
- Non-English speaking patients are at particular risk of poisoning, as the warnings on packaging of pharmaceuticals and hazardous materials can be missed.

References

Bramuzzo M, Amaddeo A, Facchina G, Neri E, Martelossi S, Barbi E. Liquid detergent capsule ingestion: a new pediatric epidemic? Pediatr Emerg Care. 2013;29(3):410–1.

Buehler MC, Gala PK, Wolfe HA, Meaney PA, Henretig FM. Laundry detergent "pod" ingestions: a case series and discussion of recent literature. Pediatr Emerg Care. 2013;29(6):743–7.

Crain EF, Gershel JC, Mezey AP. Caustic ingestions; symptoms as predictors of esophageal injury. Am J Dis Child. 1984;138(9):863–5.

Forrester MB. Comparison of pediatric exposures to concentrated "pack" and traditional laundry detergents. Pediatr Emerg Care. 2013;29(4):482–6.

Fulton JA. Caustics. In: Nelson LS, Lewis NA, Howland MA, Hoffman RS, Goldfrank LR, Flomenbaum NE, editors. Goldfrank's Toxicologic Emergencies. 9th ed. New York: McGraw-Hill; 2011. p. 1364–73.

Ng S. Safety experts raise concern over popular laundry packs—new alarm bells over single-dose detergent capsules as risk to children. The Wall Street Journal. 2013. www.wsj.com. Assessed 30 Jan 2015.

Smith E, Liebelt E, Noguiera J. Laundry detergent pod ingestions: is there a need for endoscopy? J Med Toxicol. 2014;10(3):286–91.

Valdez AL, Casavant MJ, Spiller HA, Chounthirath T, Xiang H, Smith GA. Pediatric exposure to laundry detergent pods. Pediatrics. 2014;134(6):1–9.

Williams H, Bateman N, Thomas S, Thompson J, Scott R, Vale A. Exposure to liquid detergent capsules: a study undertaken by the UK National Poison Information Service. Clin Toxicol. 2012;50(8):776–80.

Case 2
Coma and Metabolic Acidosis

1. What common xenobiotics can cause metabolic acidosis?
2. What are common industrial settings or occupations that use the substance identified?
3. What are common industrial settings or occupations that use the substance identified?
4. What is the mechanism of action of the substance identified?
5. What is the role of laboratory testing for this substance?
6. What are the cardiovascular manifestations of the substance?
7. What are potential antidotes for this substance?
8. Which occupations use this substance routinely?

Abstract Cyanide is one of the few chemicals known as a "knock down" agent, owing to its short interval from ingestion until symptom onset. In this case, a 22-year-old female attempted suicide by consuming cyanide. This chapter discusses manifestations of cyanide, diagnostic clues, and management strategies for treating acute cyanide toxicity.

Keywords Suicide • Cyanide • Metabolic acidosis • Cyanide antidote • Hydroxycobalamin

History of Present Illness

Emergency Medical Services (EMS) was called to the home of a 22-year-old female who was found unresponsive. The patient had texted a friend a suicide message 15 min prior. When the friend was not able to get in contact with the patient, the friend called EMS. EMS arrived and found the patient unresponsive.

L.R. Dye et al. (eds.), *Case Studies in Medical Toxicology*,
DOI 10.1007/978-3-319-56449-4_2

Past Medical History	Depression
Medications	Fluoxetine
Allergies	No known drug allergies
Family History	Unknown
Social History	Unknown

Physical Examination

Blood pressure	Heart rate	Respiratory rate	Temperature	O_2 saturation
80/40 mmHg	120 bpm	24 breaths/min	37 °C (98.6 °F)	98% (room air)

A suicide note and a small canister of a product purchased on-line were found near the patient.

General: Unresponsive
Cardiovascular: Regular rhythm
Pulmonary: Lungs clear bilaterally
Neuro: Intact occulocephaic reflex with normal deep tendon reflexes. Muscle tone was normal, and there was no clonus. No response to pain.

Initial Treatment

The patient was placed on a non-rebreather mask and initial labs were obtained, including a blood gas. The patient was intubated, a head CT was obtained, and an antidote was administered.

Diagnostic Testing

WBC	Hemoglobin	Platelets
14 k/mm^3	12.5 g/dL	324 k/mm^3

Na	K	Cl	CO_2	BUN	Cr	Glucose
140 mmol/L	5.5 mmol/L	105 mmol/L	8 mmol/L	14 mg/dL	1.0 mg/dL	128 mg/dL

AST	ALT
68 IU/L	41 IU/L

Acetaminophen, salicylates, and ethanol were undetectable
Arterial blood gas (FiO2: 100%): pH 7.2; PCO2: 20; PO2: 270
CarboxyHgb: 2%; MetHtb: 1%
Venous blood gas (FiO2: 100%): pH 7.19; PCO2: 21; PO2: 267

Ancillary Testing

CT head: negative for hemorrhage or masses

What Common Xenobiotics Can Cause Metabolic Acidosis?

Common xenobiotics than can cause metabolic acidosis:

• Acetaminophen	• Iron
• Acetazolamide	• Isoniazid
• Acetonitrile	• Metformin/phenformin
• Azides	• Methanol
• Carbon monoxide	• Nitroprusside
• Cyanide	• Phenol
• Didanosine	• Phosphorus
• Ethanol	• Propylene glycol
• Ethylene glycol/diethylene glycol	• Salicylates
• Ethylene glycol monobutyl ethers	• Theophylline
• Formic acid	• Toluene
• Hydrogen cyanide	• Topiramate
• Ketoacidosis (alcoholic, diabetic, etc.)	• Valproic acid

What Are Common Industrial Settings or Occupations That Use Cyanide?

Common settings and occupations that use cyanide

• Chemical manufacturing	• Metal plating
• Electroplating	• Metal stripping
• Jewelry making	• Mirror manufacturing
• Laboratory work	• Nylon production
• Metal polishing	• Pesticide manufacturing

Hospital Course

Following antidote administration, the patient's hemodynamic status improved. The patient was admitted to the intensive care unit overnight and was discharged to inpatient psychiatry 2 days later.

What Is the Mechanism of Action of Cyanide?

Cyanide inhibits numerous enzymes, especially cytochrome oxidase (Ballantyne 1987). Other enzymes inhibited by cyanide include acetoacetate decarboxylase, carbonic anhydrase, glutamic acid decarboxylase, 2-keto-4-hydroglutarate aldolase, nitrite reductase, succinate dehydrogenase, and xanthine oxidase (Curry and LoVecchio 2001). In the inner mitochondrial membrane, cyanide binds to the ferric ion in cytochrome oxidase, thereby inhibiting electron transport. As a result, adenosine triphosphate (ATP) production is profoundly inhibited. Seizures may be the result of inhibition of glutamate decarboxylase, with a subsequent decrease in GABA concentrations. In addition, cyanide stimulates the NMDA receptor (Arden et al. 1998) and increases intracellular calcium (Mathangi and Namasivayam 2004), ultimately leading to apoptosis (Mills et al. 1996).

What Is the Role of Laboratory Testing for Cyanide?

Cyanide levels can be obtained at some institutions, but are typically only performed in specialized laboratories. The levels are technically difficult to run and rarely change management, owing to long time intervals between obtaining the test and the results. There are, however, several diagnostic clues that may facilitate the diagnosis of cyanide. In the appropriate clinical setting, a lactic acid exceeding 8 mmol/L (Baud et al. 2002) (and possibly 10 mmol/L) (Huzar et al. 2013), in conjunction with a partial pressure of oxygen <10 mmHg between venous and arterial blood, may suggest the diagnosis (Gracia and Shepherd 2004).

What Are the Cardiovascular Manifestations of Cyanide?

Because the heart is particularly sensitive to ATP depletion, it is one of the most affected organs in the body. Tachycardia, with or without mild hypertension, are early findings. Later, hypotension, bradycardia, and dysrhythmias may ensue. A shortening of the ST segment can occur, resulting in a "T on R" phenomenon (Brooks et al. 2011).

What Are Potential Antidotes for Cyanide?

There are two main potential treatments for cyanide toxicity.

Historically, treatment involves a commercially available cyanide antidote kit, which contains a combination of nitrites and thiosulfate. Amyl nitrite (which is available in an inhalational ampule) and sodium nitrite (which is available intravenously as a 3% solution) can induce methemoglobinemia (Chen and Rose 1952).

The sodium nitrite is responsible for the vast majority of the nitrite production. Sodium thiosulfate serves as a sulfur donor to the enzyme rhodinase, which helps convert cyanide to thiosulfate. The typical dose of sodium nitrite is 300 mg (10 cc of a 3% solution) for adults, or 0.33 cc/kg for pediatrics. A lower dose may be utilized in anemic patients. Sodium thiosulfate is made as a 25% solution; the typical adult dose is 12.5 g (50 cc), whereas the typical pediatric dose is 1.65 cc/kg.

In cases where cyanide toxicity is felt to be present concomitantly with carbon monoxide, as may be the case in a fire victim, nitrites should be avoided due to synergistic reduction in oxygen-carrying capacity between carboxyhemoglobin and methemoglobin (Levine and Spyres 2016).

Alternatively, hydroxocobalamin, a precursor to B_{12}, can be utilized. The cobalt ion on hydroxocobalamin combines with cyanide to form cyanocobalamin (B_{12}), which is renally eliminated. The typical starting dose of hydroxocobalamin is 5 g for adults; this dose can be repeated once. Because hydroxocobalamin can produce an intense red discoloration to body fluids, laboratory parameters which rely on colormetric testing, including liver functions, creatinine, and magnesium, can be difficult to interpret (Curry et al. 1994). There is some suggestion that administration of hydroxocobalamin along with sodium thiosulfate produces synergistic effects (Rose et al. 1965).

Cobalt EDTA, which has been used in Australia and parts of Europe, chelates cyanide. The complex is then excreted in the urine (Holland and Kozlowski 1986).

In addition to antidotal therapy, crystalloid fluid boluses and direct acting vasopressors can be utilized to treat hypotension.

Which Occupations Use Cyanide Routinely?

Jewelers and those involved with precious metal reclamation are some of the more common professions to utilize cyanide. Aqueous solutions of cyanide can combine with silver or gold to form soluble compounds. Copper mines frequently have large pools of aqueous, alkaline cyanide salts to facilitate the extraction of silver and gold from impure ore (Curry and LoVecchio 2001). Cyanide is also utilized in the production of paper, plastics, rubber, mirror making, and in electroplating operations. Historically, cyanide was commonly used in photography and fumigation. While firefighters do not typically work with cyanide directly, firefighters may be exposed from cyanide through smoke inhalation.

Speciality-Specific Guidance

Prehospital

In the event of possible cyanide gas, first responders should use appropriate personal protective equipment.

Emergency Medicine

The diagnosis of cyanide toxicity should be entertained if the history suggests a rapid "knock down."

The presence of similar PO2 between the venous and arterial blood, along with a markedly elevated lactic acid (usually greater than 10), suggests the diagnosis.

Patients with concurrent elevation of carboxyhemoglobin levels should not receive nitrites, as the simultaneous generation of methemoglobinemia can be dangerous.

References

Arden SR, Sinor JD, Potthoff WK, et al. Subunit-specific interactions of cyanide with the N-methyl-D-aspartate receptor. J Biol Chem. 1998;273:21505–11.

Ballantyne B. Toxicology of cyanides. In: Ballantyne B, Marrs TC, editors. Clinical and experimental toxicology of cyanides. Bristol, England: IOP Publishing; 1987. p. 41–126.

Baud FJ, Borron SW, Megarbane B, et al. Value of lactic acidosis in the assessment of the severity of acute cyanide poisoning. Crit Care Med. 2002;30:2044–50.

Brooks DE, Levine M, O'Connor AD, et al. Toxicology in the ICU: part 2: specific toxins. Chest. 2011;140:1072–85.

Chen KK, Rose C. Nitrite and thiosulfate therapy in cyanide poisoning. JAMA. 1952;149:113–9.

Curry SC, LoVecchio FA. Hydrogen cyanide and inorganic cyanide salts. In: JB SJR, Krieger GR, editors. Clinical environmental health and toxic exposure. 2nd ed. Philadelphia, PA: Lippincott, Williams & Wilkins; 2001. p. 705–16.

Curry SC, Connor DA, Raschke RA. Effect of the cyanide antidote hydroxocobalamin on commonly ordered serum chemistry studies. Ann Emerg Med. 1994;24:65–7.

Gracia R, Shepherd G. Cyanide poisoning and its treatment. Pharmacotherapy. 2004;24:1358–65.

Holland MA, Kozlowski LM. Clinical features and management of cyanide poisoning. Clin Pharm. 1986;5:731–41.

Huzar TF, George T, Cross JM. Carbon monoxide and cyanide toxicity: etiology, pathophysiology and treatment in inhalation injury. Expert Rev Respir Med. 2013;7(2):159–70.

Levine M, Spyres M. In reply: smoke inhalation. N Engl J Med. 2016.

Mathangi DC, Namasivayam A. Calcium ions: its role in cyanide neurotoxicity. Food Chem Toxicol. 2004;42:359–61.

Mills EM, Gunasekar PG, Pavlakovic G, et al. Cyanide-induced apoptosis and oxidative stress in differentiated PC12 cells. J Neurochem. 1996;67:1039–46.

Rose CL, Worth RM, Chen KK. Hydroxo-cobalamine and acute cyanide poisoning in dogs. Life Sci. 1965;4:1785–9.

Case 3
Diet Pill Ingestion in a Child

1. What specific agents found in Mexican diet products would elicit concern for exposure?
2. Why is a diet product containing this substance concerning?
3. What is the mechanism of action of this substance?
4. What some other non-pharmaceuticals contain a substance with similar action?
5. Can you detect the presence of this non-pharmaceutical substance by obtaining a standard laboratory test?
6. When do you treat non-pharmaceutical toxicity from this substance?
7. Does an antidote reverse this non-pharmaceutical substance?
8. Why is clenbuterol used as a diet agent?
9. What are the symptoms of clenbuterol toxicity?
10. What is the mechanism of action of dinitrophenol that causes weight loss and toxicity?
11. What are the signs of dinitrophenol toxicity?

Abstract A 3-year-old male ingested several tablets of his mother's diet supplement, which had been obtained from Mexico. While he did not develop clinical signs of toxicity, exposure to this product was concerning based on the active ingredient it reportedly contained. This chapter reviews some of the agents found in "diet pills," how they cause toxicity, and clinical symptoms associated with toxicity.

Keywords Cardioselective steroids • Digoxin • *Thevetia peruviana* • Clenbuterol • Dinitrophenol

L.R. Dye et al. (eds.), *Case Studies in Medical Toxicology*,
DOI 10.1007/978-3-319-56449-4_3

History of Present Illness

A 3-year-old male was found with an open bottle of a weight loss product from Mexico. The patient's mother found him chewing on several tablets, and several tablets were found on the ground around him. On pill count, approximately 19 tablets were missing. The active ingredient listed on the weight loss agent was "troncomín 20 mg." The patient was brought to the ED 30 min after ingestion.

Past Medical History	None
Medications	None
Allergies	NKDA
Social History	Lives at home with parents and two older siblings. Mom is primary caregiver during the day
Family History	Maternal grandmother with diabetes Paternal grandfather and father with hypertension No other medical history in immediate family

Physical Examination

Blood pressure	Heart rate	Respiratory rate	Temperature	O_2 saturation	Weight
103/59 mmHg	120 bpm	16 breaths/min	37.2 °C (98.9 °F)	100% (room air)	15 kg

General: Awake, alert, sitting on mother's lap in no distress, playing and looking around room.

HEENT: Pupils were equal, round, and reactive to light. Mucus membranes were moist, normal dentition for age, no oropharyngeal erythema, edema, or ulcerations.

Cardiovascular: Regular rate; no murmurs, gallops, or rubs.

Pulmonary: Clear to auscultation bilaterally with no wheezes, rales, or rhonchi. Normal respiratory effort without stridor or accessory muscle use.

Abdomen: Soft, non-tender with no distension. Abdomen without tenderness to palpation and active bowel sounds auscultated.

Musculoskeletal: Extremities appear normal with no deformities, crepitus, or tenderness to palpation.

Skin: No clubbing or cyanosis. Warm to touch. Normal appearing skin pigment. Moist axillae.

Neurologic: Alert and will interact during exam, following basic commands. Normal muscular tone. Normal reflexes. No clonus. Face symmetric, tongue midline, and extraocular movements intact without nystagmus on direct testing.

What Specific Agents Found in Mexican Diet Products Would Elicit Concern for Exposure?

- There are several potential ingredients in Mexican diet products that are concerning. These include:
  - Yellow oleander nuts
  - Amphetamine
  - Thyroid medications
  - Dinitrophenol
  - Diuretics
  - Clenbuterol
- Commercial diet preparations from other countries may contain yellow oleander under other names: troncomín, capslim, gavafute, almendra quema grasa, *Thevetia peruviana.*

Diagnostic Testing

WBC	**Hemoglobin**	**Hematocrit**	**Platelets**	**Differential**
10 k/mm^3	12 g/dL		210 k/mm^3	

Na	**K**	**Cl**	**CO_2**	**BUN/Cr**	**Glucose**
141 mmol/L	3.5 mmol/L	105 mmol/L	24 mmol/L	8/0.3 mg/dL	103 mg/dL

Acetaminophen: negative
Salicylic acid: negative
Ethanol: negative

Ancillary Testing

EKG demonstrated sinus tachycardia with normal intervals.
Serum digoxin level 0.1 ng/mL—drawn approximately 1 h after exposure

Hospital Course

- The product ingested by the patient contained yellow oleander.
- The patient was given 1 g/kg of activated charcoal, an IV was placed, and he was transferred to a tertiary pediatric center.
- On arrival to tertiary pediatric center, his repeat vital signs were:

Blood pressure	Heart rate	Respiratory rate	Temperature	O_2 saturation
122/67 mmHg	100 bpm	15 breaths/min	37.0 °C (98.6 °F)	100% (room air)

- He was alert and exhibited age-appropriate behavior.
- A repeat digoxin level 4 h later was 0.5 ng/mL, potassium 3.7 mEq/L. His peak potassium was 4.2 mEq/L.
- The patient was admitted overnight for observation. There were no significant events on telemetry and no treatment required.
- He was discharged home the next day.

Why Is a Diet Product Containing Yellow Oleander Concerning?

- Yellow oleander contains eight different cardioactive steroids.
- Yellow oleander is a good example of a non-pharmaceutical cardioactive steroid, whereas digoxin is an example of a pharmaceutical cardioactive steroid.
- Non-pharmaceutical cardioactive steroids produce similar signs of toxicity as digoxin.
- Patients frequently experience GI symptoms and AV conduction effects as signs of toxicity after yellow oleander ingestion. However, in a large case series from Sri Lanka, very few patients developed ventricular ectopy or tachydysrhythmias (Eddleston et al. 2000a).

What Is the Mechanism of Action of Cardioactive Steroids?

- Inhibition of the Na+-K+-ATPase pump by cardioactive steroids ultimately leads to increased cytoplasmic calcium and enhances the release of calcium from the sarcoplasmic reticulum. This leads to increased strength of myocardial contraction and increased inotropy.
- Cardioactive steroids also increase vagal tone.
- In excess, cardioactive steroids may cause nonspecific symptoms such as nausea, vomiting, and abdominal pain.
- Ultimately, patients can develop bradydysrhythmias and hyperkalemia.
- AV junctional blockade is the most common dysrhythmia, but patients can also have ectopic beats and bidirectional ventricular tachycardia (Eddleston et al. 2000b)
- Hyperkalemia (>5 mEq/L) is a predictor of mortality in acute digoxin overdose. (Bismuth et al. 1973)

What Other Non-pharmaceuticals Contain Cardioactive Steroids?

- Foxglove (*Digitalis* spp)
- Oleander (*Nerium oleander*)
- Lilly of the valley (*Convallaria majalis*)
- Red squill (*Urginea maritima*)
- *Bufo* species of frogs

Can You Detect the Presence of Non-pharmaceutical Cardioactive Steroids by Obtaining a Standard Digoxin Level?

- Some immunoassays for digoxin cross-react with these compounds (Barrueto et al. 2003).
- Other assays are more specific for pharmaceutical digoxin and may not cross-react. Specifically, there are reports of monoclonal assays that do not detect non-pharmaceutical cardioactive steroids (Brubacher et al. 1996; Dasgupta 2004).
- Digoxin levels in these cases are helpful as a dichotomous positive/negative test, **but actual levels do not predict degree of toxicity** (Dasgupta 2006)

When Do You Treat Non-pharmaceutical Cardioactive Steroid Toxicity?

- It is reasonable to give patients with acute/accidental ingestions a single dose of activated charcoal in an effort to prevent absorption of cardioactive steroids. Additionally, there is evidence of enterohepatic recirculation of these compounds and multi-dose activated charcoal may be warranted in some cases to enhance elimination.
- Initially, activated charcoal can be given, if warranted. IV access, cardiac monitoring, and frequent electrolytes are warranted.
- The utility of repeating digoxin levels is unknown as these are not direct measures of the circulating non-pharmaceutical cardioactive steroid, but rather a cross-reaction between this and the digoxin assay (Dasgupta 2006).
- Consider digoxin-specific Fab fragments (DigiBind or DigiFab) for patients with a potassium >5 mEq/L **symptomatic** bradycardia, increased automaticity and ectopy, or ventricular dysrhythmias (Lapostolle et al. 2008).
- Consider conservative observation for asymptomatic patients with non-pharmaceutical cardioactive steroid ingestion.
- The aggressiveness of the approach to treatment may be different with chronic toxicity/chronic use of these products—but ultimately will be patient-dependent.

Do Digoxin-Specific Fab Fragments Work in the Reversal of Non-pharmaceutical Cardioactive Steroid Toxicity?

- There are several studies and case reports that describe efficacy of digoxin-specific Fab fragments in the treatment of plant cardiac glycosides and bufadienolide toxicity (Cheung et al. 1991; Barrueto et al. 2003; Brubacher et al. 1996, 1999; Eddleston et al. 2000a; Safadi et al. 1995).
- Patients with toxicity from non-pharmaceutical cardioactive steroids may require much higher doses of digoxin-specific Fab fragments and repeated dosing for stabilization (up to 37 vials has been described) due to decreased affinity of digoxin fab for non-pharmaceutical cardioactive steroids (Rich et al. 1993).
- 10–20 vials of digoxin-specific Fab fragments are recommended as the initial starting dose for patients with clinical signs of digoxin-like toxicity from non-pharmaceutical cardioactive steroids. (Barrueto et al. 2003; Safadi et al. 1995)

Why Is Clenbuterol Used as a Diet Agent?

- Clenbuterol is a β2 agonist that increases causing muscle hypertrophy and the growth of fast-twitch muscle fibers.
- It is used in cattle to increase the amount of muscle and decrease fat.

What Are Symptoms of Clenbuterol Toxicity?

- Tachycardia (Ramos et al. 2004)
- Nausea and diarrhea (Ramos et al. 2004)
- Tremors (Ramos et al. 2004)
- Hypertension (Ramos et al. 2004)
- Leukocytosis (Ramos et al. 2004)
- Hypokalemia (Ramos et al. 2004)

What Is the Mechanism of Action of Dinitrophenol That Causes Weight Loss and Toxicity?

- Dinitrophenol (2,4-dinitrophenol) increases metabolic activity by uncoupling oxidative phosphorylation.
- By uncoupling oxidative phosphorylation, ATP cannot be synthesized in the mitochondria.
- The energy that normally goes into creating the bond between ADP and phosphate is dissipated as heat causing profound hyperthermia.

What Are Signs of Dinitrophenol Toxicity?

- Hyperthermia
- Agranulocytosis
- Diaphoresis
- Increased thirst
- Respiratory failure
- Malaise
- Skin rash
- Coma
- Death

Case Conclusion

In this case, a 3-year-old male was exposed to a Mexican diet aid, which contained yellow oleander (*Thevetia peruviana*). Herbal and supplement-based diet aids have been associated with many different toxicities including clenbuterol, 2,4-dinitrophenol, and non-pharmaceutical cardiac glycoside toxicity. This patient was given activated charcoal and observed overnight. He required no additional treatment and did not develop signs of clinical toxicity even though exposure was likely, given the positive digoxin assay.

Specialty-Specific Guidance

Internal Medicine/Family Medicine

- Digoxin levels may help detect exposure to non-pharmaceutical cardioactive steroids, but levels do not correlate with toxicity. As assays become more specific for digoxin, there will be less cross-reactivity with other cardioactive steroids. A negative lab value does not rule out exposure, and the utility of repeated digoxin levels is unknown.
- Obtain electrolytes and initial EKG for all patients with suspected exposure.
- Most patients with accidental/intentional acute ingestions will require observation, telemetry monitoring for signs of toxicity and consultation with a toxicologist or poison center.
- EKG findings of bidirectional ventricular tachycardia are nearly diagnostic of cardioactive steroid exposure, whether via digoxin or non-pharmaceutical cardiac glycosides.
- Key features of toxicity include: hyperkalemia, symptomatic bradycardia, and a variety of dysrhythmias.
- As with digoxin toxicity, repeat digoxin levels should not be obtained once Fab fragments have been administered. Additional dosing of digoxin-specific Fab fragments should be based on clinical symptoms.

Pediatrics

- Digoxin levels may help detect exposure to non-pharmaceutical cardioactive steroids, but levels do not correlate with toxicity. As assays become more specific for digoxin, there will be less cross-reactivity with other cardioactive steroids. A negative lab value does not rule out exposure, and the utility of repeated digoxin levels is unknown.
- Obtain electrolytes and initial EKG for all patients with suspected exposure.
- Most patients with accidental/intentional acute ingestions will require observation, telemetry monitoring for signs of toxicity and consultation with a toxicologist or poison center.
- EKG findings of bidirectional ventricular tachycardia are nearly diagnostic of cardioactive steroid exposure, whether via digoxin or non-pharmaceutical cardiac glycosides.
- Key features of toxicity include: hyperkalemia, symptomatic bradycardia, and a variety of dysrhythmias.
- As with digoxin toxicity, repeat digoxin levels should not be obtained once Fab fragments have been administered. Additional dosing of digoxin-specific Fab fragments should be based on clinical symptoms.

Emergency Medicine

- Consider activated charcoal to prevent absorption of recently ingested cardioactive steroids, especially if the patient presents within 1 h of ingestion.
- There are some cases where multi-dose activated charcoal may be recommended as many cardioactive steroids (pharmaceutical and non-pharmaceutical) are reported to have enterohepatic recirculation.
- Digoxin levels may detect exposure to a non-pharmaceutical cardioactive steroid, but levels do not correlate with toxicity. As assays become more specific for digoxin, there will be less cross-reactivity with other cardioactive steroids. A negative lab value does not mean a lack of exposure, and the utility of obtaining repeated digoxin levels is unknown.
- Obtain electrolytes and initial EKG for all patients with suspected exposure.
- Most patients with accidental/intentional acute ingestions will require observation, telemetry monitoring for signs of toxicity, and consultation with a toxicologist or poison center.
- An EKG demonstrating bidirectional ventricular tachycardia is nearly diagnostic of cardioactive steroid exposure, whether via digoxin or non-pharmaceutical cardiac glycosides.
- Patients with toxicity from non-pharmaceutical cardioactive steroids may require much higher doses of digoxin-specific Fab fragments for stabilization due to decreased affinity of digoxin fab for non-pharmaceutical cardioactive steroids. An initial recommended dose is 10–20 vials.

- As with digoxin toxicity, repeat digoxin levels should not be obtained once Fab fragments have been administered. Additional dosing of digoxin-specific Fab fragments should be based on the patient's clinical symptoms.

Toxicology

- Consider activated charcoal to prevent absorption of recently ingested cardioactive steroids, especially if the patient presents within 1 h of ingestion.
- There are some cases where multi-dose activated charcoal may be recommended as many cardioactive steroids (pharmaceutical and non-pharmaceutical) are reported to have enterohepatic recirculation.
- Digoxin levels may detect exposure to a non-pharmaceutical cardioactive steroid, but levels do not correlate with toxicity. As assays become more specific for digoxin, there will be less cross-reactivity with other cardioactive steroids. A negative lab value does not rule out exposure, and the utility of obtaining repeated digoxin levels is unknown.
- Obtain electrolytes and initial EKG for all patients with suspected exposure.
- Most patients with accidental/intentional acute ingestions will require observation and telemetry monitoring for signs of toxicity.
- An EKG demonstrating bidirectional ventricular tachycardia is nearly diagnostic of cardioactive steroid exposure, whether via digoxin or non-pharmaceutical cardiac glycosides.
- Patients with toxicity from non-pharmaceutical cardioactive steroids may require much higher doses of digoxin-specific Fab fragments for stabilization due to decreased affinity of digoxin fab for non-pharmaceutical cardioactive steroids. An initial recommended dose is 10–20 vials.
- As with digoxin toxicity, repeat digoxin levels should not be obtained once Fab fragments have been administered. Additional dosing of digoxin-specific Fab fragments should be based on the patient's clinical symptoms.

References

Bismuth C, Gaultier M, Conso F, Efthymiou M. Hyperkalemia in acute digitalis poisoning: prognostic significance and therapeutic implications. Clin Toxicol. 1973;6:153–62.

Barrueto F, Jortani S, Valdes R, Hoffman R, Nelson L. Cardioactive steroid poisoning from an herbal cleansing preparation. Ann Emerg Med. 2003;41:396–9.

Brubacher J, Hoffman R, Kile T. Toad venom poisoning: failure of a monoclonal digoxin immune assay to cross-react with the cardioactive steroids. Clin Toxicol. 1996;34(5):529–30.

Brubacher J, Lachmanen D, Ravikumar P, Hoffman R. Efficacy of digoxin specific Fab fragments (Digibind®) in the treatment of toad venom poisoning. Toxicon. 1999;37:931–42.

Cheung K, Urech R, Taylor L, Duffy P, Radford D. Plant cardiac glycosides and digoxine Fab antibody. J Paediatr Child Health. 1991;27(5):312–3.

Dasgupta A. Therapeutic drug monitoring of digoxin: impact of endogenous and exogenous digoxin-like immunoreactive substances. Toxicol Rev. 2006;25:273–81.

Dasgupta A, Datta P. Rapid detection of oleander poisoning using digoxin immunoassays: comparison of five assays. Ther Drug Monit. 2004;26(6):658–63.

Eddleston M, Rajapakse S, Rajakanthan K, et al. Anti-digoxin Fab fragments in cardiotoxicity induced by ingestion of yellow oleander: a randomized controlled trial. Lancet. 2000a;355(9208):967–72.

Eddleston M, Ariaratnam C, Sjostrom L, et al. Acute yellow oleander (Thevetia peruviana) poisoning: cardiac arrhythmias, electrolyte disturbances, and serum cardiac glycoside concentrations on presentation to hospital. Heart. 2000b;83:301–6.

Lapostolle F, et al. Digoxin-specific Fab fragments as single first-line therapy in digitalis poisoning. Crit Care Med. 2008;36:3014–8.

Ramos F, Silveira I, Silva JM, et al. Proposed guidelines for clenbuterol food poisoning. Am J Med. 2004;117:362.

Rich SA, Libera JM, Locke RJ. Treatment of foxglove extract poisoning with digoxin-specific Fab fragments. Ann Emerg Med. 1993;22:1904–7.

Safadi R, Levy I, Amitai Y, Caraco Y. Beneficial effect of digoxin-specific Fab fragments in oleander intoxication. Arch Intern Med. 1995;155:2121–5.

Case 4
Salicylate Ingestion

1. What are the sources of salicylates?
2. What are the signs and symptoms of acute salicylate toxicity?
3. What are the pharmacokinetics of salicylates?
4. What laboratory tests are useful in acute salicylate toxicity?
5. How are salicylate levels measured and reported?
6. What acid-base disturbances can be expected in acute salicylate toxicity?
7. What effects on coagulation are possible?
8. What is the role of activated charcoal?
9. What is the role of intravenous fluid resuscitation?
10. What is the rationale for sodium bicarbonate therapy?
11. How can declining salicylate levels be interpreted?
12. What are the indications for extracorporeal removal (hemodialysis)?
13. How does chronic salicylate toxicity differ?

Abstract Salicylate, widely available and most commonly encountered as acetylsalicylic acid (Aspirin®), may cause rapidly fatal toxicity. Clinical manifestations of salicylate poisoning include gastrointestinal symptoms, tinnitus, coagulopathy, severe metabolic disturbances, uncoupling of oxidative phosphorylation, pulmonary edema, and central nervous system toxicity including encephalopathy, seizures, coma, cerebral edema, and death. We report a case of a 47-year-old man with intentional salicylate ingestion. Sources of salicylate, clinical effects of the drug, and diagnostic testing strategies are reviewed. We describe appropriate treatment options and the indications for treatment of salicylate poisoning, including gastrointestinal decontamination, fluid resuscitation, alkaline therapy with sodium bicarbonate, and extracorporeal removal via hemodialysis.

Keywords Salicylate • Aspirin® • Poisoning • Ingestion • Toxicity • Acidosis • Alkalinization

L.R. Dye et al. (eds.), *Case Studies in Medical Toxicology*,
DOI 10.1007/978-3-319-56449-4_4

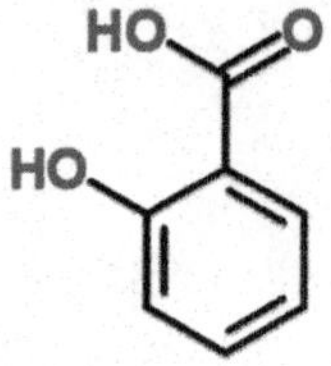

Emergency Department

Chief Complaint: Tinnitus, nausea, vomiting.

History of Present Illness

A 47-year-old man was brought to the ED from his group home by EMS for ringing in the ears, nausea, and vomiting for approximately 16 h. He reported ingesting over 300 enteric-coated baby aspirin (81 mg) more than 24 h prior in a suicide attempt. He denied shortness of breath, chest pain, palpitations, diarrhea, confusion, weakness, numbness, tingling, or urinary complaints.

What Are Sources of Salicylates?

The bark of the willow tree has historically been used for anti-inflammatory and analgesic properties. Willow bark extract (salicin) is marketed as an over-the-counter herbal alternative to aspirin. After oral absorption of salicin, some salicylic acid is produced as a metabolite, but typically not in sufficient quantity to be a source of toxicity (Schmid et al. 2001).

Due to the irritating effects of oral salicylic acid, research continued and led to the marketing of acetylsalicylic acid as Aspirin®. Salicylic acid is now primarily used topically as a keratolytic. Due to slower dermal absorption, toxicity is less common, although possible (Brubacher and Hoffman 1996). Currently, acetylsalicylic acid is the most common source of salicylate and is available in multiple formulations including tablet, chewable, enteric-coated, controlled-release, suppository, and liquid forms.

Methyl salicylate is another form that is found in topical rubefacients like Bengay® or Icy Hot®, but transdermal toxicity is uncommon due to slow absorption. However, if a cream is ingested, absorption is greater and can pose a risk (Wolowich et al. 2003). From a toxicological standpoint, the most concerning source of methyl salicylate is oil of wintergreen (*Gaultheria procumbens*). One milliliter of 98% oil of wintergreen contains the equivalent of a 1.4 g dose of aspirin, making a teaspoon more than enough to kill a toddler (Vandenberg et al. 1989). Many other methyl salicylate glycosides are found in a variety of plants and there is active research into potential uses (Mao et al. 2014).

Bismuth subsalicylate (active ingredient in Pepto-Bismol®) contains the equivalent of 8.7 mg of salicylic acid in 1 mL and can lead to salicylate toxicity as well, though typically with chronic use (Sainsbury 1991).

Emergency Department (Continued)

Past Medical History	Mild Intellectual disability Hypertension Schizophrenia Obsessive-compulsive disorder
Medications	Sertraline 100 mg PO daily Clozapine 100 mg PO qHS Buspirone 15 mg PO BID Haloperidol 100 mg IM q 4 weeks Lithium carbonate 300 mg PO qAM + 600 mg qPM Docusate 100 mg PO BID
Allergies	NKDA
Family History	Reviewed and non-contributory
Social History	Smokes 1 pack per day, denies alcohol use, smokes marijuana weekly. Lives in a group setting with other behavioral health patients

Physical Examination

Blood pressure	**Heart rate**	**Respiratory rate**	**Temperature**	**O_2 saturation**
122/83 mmHg	122 bpm	22 (deep)	36.6 °C (97.88 °F)	98% (room air)

General: Awake in bed. Cooperative with exam. Answering all questions appropriately.

HENT: Normocephalic. Moist mucous membranes.

Eyes: Pupils 4 mm and reactive bilaterally. Extra-ocular movements intact.

Resp: No respiratory distress, but tachypneic and hyperpneic. Lung sounds clear to auscultation.

CV: Tachycardic without murmurs, rubs, or gallops.

GI/Abd: Soft, mild LUQ/epigastric tenderness. No rebound or guarding.

Musculoskeletal: No swelling, tenderness, or deformity.

Skin: Warm and dry. No rashes.

Neuro: Alert and oriented to person, place, and time. Cranial nerves 2–12 intact except diminished hearing (to finger-rub) bilaterally. Moving all extremities. Grossly normal sensation. Normal muscle tone. No clonus.

What Are Signs and Symptoms of Acute Salicylate Toxicity?

Early manifestations of acute salicylate toxicity include nausea and vomiting, likely due to both direct irritation and chemoreceptor trigger zone stimulation. Epigastric discomfort can occur from irritation and pylorospasm that, along with bezoar formation, can delay absorption. Hearing is commonly affected with both tinnitus (Puel 2007) and hearing loss (Kakehata and Santos-Sacchi 1996) via independent mechanisms. Finally, an important sign is a change in respiratory rate and depth because of direct stimulation of the central respiratory center, as well as increased carbon dioxide production secondary to uncoupling of oxidative phosphorylation. Uncoupling also leads to elevated body temperature as energy from cellular respiration is released as heat.

What Are the Pharmacokinetics of Salicylates?

Salicylates are well-absorbed orally. However, depending on the product type, absorption can be delayed, as suggested in this case, and kinetics can be erratic in overdose (Leonards and Levy 1965). Dermal absorption is slower, but can reach toxic levels under conditions that would be expected to increase skin absorption (non-intact skin, warm skin, etc.). Salicylates bind to albumin and increasing salicylate levels will saturate protein binding causing free salicylate levels to increase.

Salicylates are metabolized by the liver to salicyluric acid and conjugated with glycine and glucuronide; these products are then renally eliminated in the urine. Normal metabolic pathways are saturable with ingestions as small as a single aspirin dose of 300 mg (Bedford et al. 1965). As normal metabolic pathways become saturated, salicylate elimination changes from *first-order* to *zero-order* elimination. Importantly, the volume of distribution of salicylate also increases significantly with rising serum salicylate concentrations or falling blood pH, increasing the proportion of drug in the tissues, and thus, toxicity.

What Laboratory Tests Are Useful in Acute Salicylate Toxicity?

A basic metabolic panel (BMP) will provide information about electrolytes, metabolic acid-base balance, and renal function. A blood gas will help determine overall acid-base status and guide alkaline therapy. Serial serum salicylate levels help to guide ongoing therapy and termination of treatment.

How Are Salicylate Levels Measured and Reported?

Salicylate levels are commonly measured using Trinder's colorimetric assay in which ferric (Fe^{3+}) ions react with salicylates to form a purple compound. Using a spectrophotometer, the optical density is then measured at 540 nm (Trinder 1954). Not surprisingly, other substances that absorb at this wavelength can interfere with this assay. This includes medications such as diflunisal (also known as 5-(2,4-difluorophenyl)salicylic acid), phenothiazines, and even acetylcysteine. Hyperbilirubinemia can also falsely elevate levels using this assay (Berkovitch et al. 2000). Immunoassays using fluorescence polarization are not affected by bilirubin or phenothiazines.

In the United States, serum salicylate levels can be reported in a variety of units depending on the lab. Attention to units is crucial for appropriate management decisions (1 mg/dL = 10 μg/mL). Therapeutic levels are generally less than 20 mg/dL.

Diagnostic Testing

WBC	Hemoglobin	Hematocrit	Platelets
15.5 k/mm^3	15.5 g/dL	42.5%	336 k/mm^3

Na	K	Cl	CO_2	BUN	Cr	Glucose
140 mmol/L	3.8 mmol/L	117 mmol/L	18 mmol/L	10 mg/dL	1.1 mg/dL	107 mg/dL

Salicylate: 68.5 mg/dL (reference range: 4–20 mg/dL)
Magnesium: 2.4 mg/dL (reference range: 1.7–2.4 mg/dL)
Prothrombin Time: 17.2 s (reference range: 11.8–14.7 s)
VBG: pH: 7.49, PCO_2: 24, PO_2: 31
Urine pH: 6.0

What Acid-Base Disturbances Can Be Expected in Acute Salicylate Toxicity?

The increased minute ventilation discussed above leads to respiratory alkalosis as demonstrated in this patient. As toxicity progresses, an anion gap metabolic acidosis develops due to several factors:

(a) salicylic acid and its metabolites

(b) decreased aerobic metabolism leading to increased organic acids (e.g., pyruvic, lactic, and acetoacetic acids)
(c) decreased renal function leading to sulfuric and phosphoric acid build-up

What Effects on Coagulation Are Possible?

Acetylsalicylic acid irreversibly impairs platelet function (Schafer 1995). Salicylates can increase prothrombin time (PT); the proposed mechanism is inhibition of production of Vitamin K-dependent coagulation factors (Joss and LeBlond 2000).

Initial Treatment

The patient received bolus IV crystalloids during transport by EMS. In the ED, he received a bolus of 8.4% sodium bicarbonate 100 mEq IV and then was started on a sodium bicarbonate drip (sodium bicarbonate 150 mEq + KCl 40 mEq in 1 L of D5W) at 200 mL/h (~1.75 × calculated maintenance rate).

What Is the Role of Activated Charcoal?

Awake, alert, cooperative patients presenting within 1 h of ingestion may be given activated charcoal, if tolerated (Curtis et al. 1984). Multiple doses of activated charcoal have also been demonstrated to reduce the absorption of salicylate in experimental models (Barone et al. 1988). In cases with ongoing absorption despite appropriate management, more than one dose of activated charcoal may be considered, but must be balanced against the risk of aspiration. However, no study has demonstrated an improvement in patient-centered outcomes with the use of single or multiple-dose activated charcoal in salicylate poisoning (American Academy of Clinical Toxicology 1999).

What Is the Role of Intravenous Fluid Resuscitation?

Patients with salicylate toxicity are generally volume-depleted due to a variety of factors including vomiting and increased insensible losses. Replenishing volume, as opposed to over-hydration, is the appropriate goal. Potassium replacement prevents renal resorption of potassium in exchange for protons and subsequent failure of urinary alkalinization.

What Is the Rationale for Sodium Bicarbonate Therapy?

Acetylsalicylic acid is a weak acid with $pK_a = 3.5$ at 25 °C (77 °F). Under alkaline conditions, the deprotonated, or ionized, form increases. This charged form crosses cell membranes less efficiently and thus can accumulate in an alkaline environment. By alkalinizing serum, diffusion of acetylsalicylic acid out of blood can be decreased which in turn protects the brain. Alkalinization of urine attempts to trap ionized salicylate and enhance elimination. Typical goals for alkaline therapy are a serum pH between 7.5–7.55 and urine pH of 8. Aggressive ongoing replacement of potassium is critical to achieve urinary alkalinization, as renal acidification of urine will occur in a potassium-avid state.

Is It Safe to Intubate Patients with Salicylate Toxicity?

Anecdote and case reports have promulgated the idea that endotracheal intubation is, by nature, deleterious in patients with salicylate poisoning. Some authors have gone so far as to suggest that intubation be withheld until cardiopulmonary arrest has occurred (Greenberg et al. 2003). It is true that intubation is a potentially dangerous event in a salicylate-poisoned patient because decreasing pH increases the effective volume of distribution of salicylate and allows un-ionized salicylate into the central nervous system where lethal toxicity may occur. However, there is no evidence in the literature that intubation causes intrinsic harm, nor that it should be withheld in a patient who requires intubation based on accepted indications such as failure to oxygenate, failure to ventilate, or loss of airway protective reflexes. Attention must be paid to accomplishing intubation as rapidly as possible, with the minimum reduction in minute ventilation and the shortest possible apnea time. Initial ventilator settings should attempt to match or exceed the patient's minute ventilation at the time of induction and arterial blood gases rapidly obtained thereafter so that ventilator settings and treatment can be appropriately titrated and acidosis prevented (Bora and Aaron 2010).

Hospital Course

The patient was admitted to the ICU by the inpatient toxicology service. His sodium bicarbonate drip was continued. A blood gas and urine pH were repeated to confirm appropriate alkalinization; serial BMP and salicylate levels were obtained to guide continued therapy. Once the salicylate level decreased to less than 25 mg/dL, the bicarbonate drip was stopped, and the salicylate level rechecked 4 h later to verify continued decline. All of his symptoms resolved and he was discharged to behavioral health.

How Can Declining Salicylate Levels Be Interpreted?

Ideally, declining serum salicylate levels would indicate effective elimination and a decreasing body burden of the drug. However, it is important to consider the patient's clinical condition because levels can also decline from redistribution out of blood and into body tissues, the most concerning of which would be accumulation in the central nervous system. In fact, serum salicylate levels among those who die of salicylate poisoning are similar to those among patients who recover (Chapman and Proudfoot 1989).

What Are the Indications for Extracorporeal Removal (Hemodialysis)?

The Extracorporeal Treatments in Poisoning (EXTRIP) working group recommends hemodialysis for clinical evidence of severe toxicity (central nervous system toxicity, acute respiratory distress syndrome, or refractory acid-base or electrolyte disturbances) on the basis of level 1D evidence. EXTRIP further recommends hemodialysis for all patients with salicylate level > 100 mg/dL, regardless of signs or symptoms, and for those with level > 90 mg/dL in the setting of renal impairment (Juurlink et al. 2015). Medical conditions that prevent adequate alkalinization due to limitations on volume administration (e.g., congestive heart failure) may also warrant hemodialysis. Hemodialysis is preferred over continuous renal replacement therapies because of the higher drug clearance that can be achieved through hemodialysis. Charcoal hemoperfusion is acceptable if hemodialysis is unavailable, but most facilities now lack the capacity to perform this treatment. Hemodialysis should also be considered in cases of chronic toxicity with concerning symptoms.

How Does Chronic Salicylate Toxicity Differ?

Patients have similar symptoms as in acute toxicity, but serum levels are often much lower. Recognition is often delayed because of the insidious onset of symptoms that may mimic other common conditions, such as diabetic ketoacidosis or delirium. Early recognition is critical, as in-hospital mortality of chronic salicylism has been reported to increase threefold if the diagnosis is delayed beyond the emergency department (O'Malley 2007). It is important to consider chronic salicylism and order a salicylate level, even in the absence of ingestion or overdose history, in an elderly patient without a clear cause for metabolic acidosis or neurologic deterioration (Durnas and Cusack 1992).

Specialty-Specific Guidance

Prehospital

- Any claim of salicylate ingestion, especially if in an attempt at self-harm, should be taken seriously and transported for further evaluation.
- Fluid resuscitation is important to replace lost volume.
- If intubation is required, attempts should be made to preserve the patient's minute ventilation; avoid prolonged apnea and respiratory acidosis, which worsen toxicity.

Emergency Medicine

- As for prehospital.
- Sodium bicarbonate for serum and urine alkalinization to goal pH 7.5–7.55 and 8, respectively.
- Potassium must be replaced to permit adequate urinary alkalinization.
- Serial blood gases, salicylate levels, and metabolic panels help guide management.
- Hemodialysis is indicated for central nervous system toxicity, refractory acid-base or electrolyte disturbances, or oliguric/anuric acute renal failure.

Critical Care Medicine

- Hyperthermia is a sign of uncoupling of oxidative phosphorylation and is associated with a poor prognosis.
- Hemodialysis is indicated for central nervous system toxicity, refractory acid-base or electrolyte disturbances, or oliguric/anuric acute renal failure.
- Continue bicarbonate for alkalinization until serum salicylate level is less than 25 mg/dL.
- Monitor serial salicylate levels and electrolytes as well as blood gas and urine pH as necessary.
- Recheck salicylate level after alkalinization has stopped to ensure level continues to decline.

References

American Academy of Clinical Toxicology, European Association of Poisons Centres and Clinical Toxicologists. Position statement and practice guidelines on the use of multi-dose activated charcoal in the treatment of acute poisoning. J Toxicol Clin Toxicol. 1999;37(6):731–51.

Barone JA, Raia JJ, Huang YC. Evaluation of the effects of multiple-dose activated charcoal on the absorption of orally administered salicylate in a simulated toxic ingestion model. Ann Emerg Med. 1988;17(1):34–7.

Bedford C, Cummings AJ, Martin BK. A kinetic study of the elimination of salicylate in man. Br J Pharmacol Chemother. 1965;24:418–31.

Berkovitch M, Uziel Y, Greenberg R, Chen-Levy Z, Arcusin M, Marcus O, Pinto O, Evans S, Matias A, Lahat E. False-high blood salicylate levels in neonates with hyperbilirubinemia. Ther Drug Monit. 2000;22(6):757–61.

Bora K, Aaron C. Pitfalls in salicylate toxicity. Am J Emerg Med. 2010;28(3):383–4.

Brubacher JR, Hoffman RS. Salicylism from topical salicylates: review of the literature. J Toxicol Clin Toxicol. 1996;34(4):431–6.

Chapman BJ, Proudfoot AT. Adult salicylate poisoning: deaths and outcome in patients with high plasma salicylate concentrations. The Quarterly Journal of Medicine. 1989;72(268):699–707.

Curtis RA, Barone J, Giacona N. Efficacy of ipecac and activated charcoal/cathartic. Prevention of salicylate absorption in a simulated overdose. Arch Intern Med. 1984;144(1):48–52.

Durnas C, Cusack BJ. Salicylate intoxication in the elderly. Recognition and recommendations on how to prevent it. Drugs Aging. 1992;2(1):20–34.

Greenberg MI, Hendrickson RG, Hofman M. Deleterious effects of endotracheal intubation in salicylate poisoning. Ann Emerg Med. 2003;41(4):583–4.

Joss JD, LeBlond RF. Potentiation of warfarin anticoagulation associated with topical methyl salicylate. The Annals of Pharmacotherapy. 2000;34(6):729–33.

Juurlink DN, Gosselin S, Kielstein JT, Ghannoum M, Lavergne V, Nolin TD, Hoffman RS. Extracorporeal treatment for salicylate poisoning: systematic review and recommendations from the EXTRIP workgroup. Ann Emerg Med. 2015;66(2):165–81.

Kakehata S, Santos-Sacchi J. Effects of salicylate and lanthanides on outer hair cell motility and associated gating charge. J Neurosci. 1996;16(16):4881–9.

Leonards JR, Levy G. Absorption and metabolism of aspirin administered in enteric-coated tablets. JAMA. 1965;193:99–104.

Mao P, Liu Z, Xie M, Jiang R, Liu W, Wang X, Meng S, She G. Naturally occurring methyl salicylate glycosides. Mini Rev Med Chem. 2014;14(1):56–63.

O'Malley GF. Emergency department management of the salicylate-poisoned patient. Emerg Med Clin North Am. 2007;25(2):333–46; abstract viii.

Puel JL. Cochlear NMDA receptor blockade prevents salicylate-induced tinnitus. B-ENT. 2007;3(Suppl 7):19–22.

Sainsbury SJ. Fatal salicylate toxicity from bismuth subsalicylate. West J Med. 1991;155(6):637–9.

Schmid B, Kötter I, Heide L. Pharmacokinetics of salicin after oral administration of a standardised willow bark extract. Eur J Clin Pharmacol. 2001;57(5):387–91.

Schafer AI. Effects of non steroidal antiinflammatory drugs on platelet function and systemic hemostasis. J Clin Pharmacol. 1995;35(3):209–19.

Trinder P. Rapid determination of salicylate in biological fluids. Biochem J. 1954;57(2):301–3.

Vandenberg SA, Smolinske SC, Spoerke DG, Rumack BH. Non-aspirin salicylates: conversion factors for estimating aspirin equivalency. Vet Hum Toxicol. 1989;31(1):49–50.

Wolowich WR, Hadley CM, Kelley MT, Walson PD, Casavant MJ. Plasma salicylate from methyl salicylate cream compared to oil of wintergreen. J Toxicol Clin Toxicol. 2003;41(4):355–8.

Case 5
Exotic Snake Envenomation

1. What is your differential diagnosis if this case takes place in the US?
2. How does the differential diagnosis change if this case takes place in Australia?
3. Which Australian snakes cause neurotoxicity or coagulopathy? Which snakes cause both?
4. How does the coral snake venom cause neurotoxicity and how does the clinical presentation differ between the two coral snakes found in the US?
5. How does botulism toxin produce neurologic symptoms?
6. What venoms are tested for with the Australian snake venom detection kit, also called the CSL™ SVDK (CSL 2007)?
7. What specimens can be used to test for venom with the snake venom detection kit, which can only be used for detecting Australian snake envenomations?
8. There are two types of antivenin (AV) available in Australia for envenomation by this snake, polyvalent and monovalent. What is the difference between the two types of antivenin?
9. Why is monovalent antivenin a better choice for treatment of envenomation by this snake?
10. When should antivenin (AV) be given in envenomations by this snake? What is the recommended dose?
11. Why would neostigmine be considered for use in this patient?
12. Where do the toxins from the venom from this Australasia snake act?
13. What does this snake look like? What features distinguish it from other venomous snakes in Australasia?
14. What are the indications for a pressure immobilization bandage (PIB)? How does one apply it on a bitten patient? What are the potential pros and cons of PIB?
15. What are some of the acute and longer-term adverse effects of snake antivenin administration?

L.R. Dye et al. (eds.), *Case Studies in Medical Toxicology*,
DOI 10.1007/978-3-319-56449-4_5

Abstract In this case, a patient is envenomated by his friend's exotic pet snake. The patient rapidly develops signs of neurotoxicity, including blurred vision, ptosis, and difficulty swallowing. He ultimately develops respiratory arrest and bradycardia. In this chapter, we review some of the toxins that can cause progressive neurologic symptoms including botulinum toxin, neurotoxic snakes in the US, and some of the exotic snakes that can cause neurologic effects.

Keywords Envenomation • Neurologic dysfunction • Respiratory depression • Coral snake • Death adder • Botulism

History of Present Illness

20-year-old male was housesitting for a friend and feeding his friend's pet snake when the snake grabbed and bit his middle finger. He had nausea, vomited twice, and wrapped a constriction bandage around his right arm. He presented to the Emergency Department within 30 min of envenomation and complained of blurred vision on arrival.

Past Medical History	Asthma
Medications	Salbutamol as needed
Allergies	NKDA
Social History	Denies tobacco use Occasional alcohol consumption No other drug use

Physical Examination

Blood pressure	Heart rate	Respiratory rate	O_2 saturation
150/90 mmHg	113 bpm	18 breaths/min	100% (room air)

General: The patient was awake and alert.
Cardiovascular: Tachycardia with normal distal pulses and no murmurs, gallops, or rubs
Pulmonary: Normal respiratory rate without stridor or accessory muscle use noted. No wheezing, rales, or rhonci
Skin: Local signs at the bite site included a double puncture wound with no swelling or redness. There was no evidence of bleeding at bite site.
Neurologic: Examination was significant for ptosis, blurred vision, difficulty swallowing, and loss of gag reflex. He had normal muscular tone, reflexes, and strength on direct testing of his upper and lower limbs. No ophthalmoplegia was noted.

What Is Your Differential Diagnosis If This Case Takes Place in the US?

- Coral snake
- Mojave rattlesnake
- Imported snake envenomation with neurotoxic venom
- Consider other diagnoses unrelated to the snake bite
- Botulism
- Myasthenia gravis
- Buckthorn (*Karwinskia humboldtiana*) poisoning
- Paralytic shellfish poisoning
- Hypermagnesemia

How Does the Differential Diagnosis Change If This Case Takes Place in Australia?

- Need to consider Brown snake, Tiger snake, Taipan, and death adder envenomations if this case occurs in Australia.

Which Australian Snakes Cause Neurotoxicity or Coagulopathy? Which Snakes Cause Both?

Snake	Coagulopathy	Neurotoxicity
Brown snake	+++	–
Tiger snake	+++	++
Taipan	+++	+++
Death adder	–	+++

Note that this is a simplified table—a more comprehensive table can be found in Isbister et al. 2013

How Does the Coral Snake Venom Cause Neurotoxicity and How Does the Clinical Presentation Differ Between the Two Coral Snakes Found in the US?

- *Micrurus fulvius* (Eastern coral snake) and *Micrurus tener* (Texas coral snake) are the two types of coral snakes found in the US with neurotoxic venom effects (Norris 2009).
- Effects from *M. fulvius* envenomation tend to be more severe than those noted with *M. tener* envenomation.
- *M. fulvius* venom has components that interfere with post-synaptic acetylcholine receptors causing neuromuscular blockade and paralysis (Weiss and McIsaac 1971; Snyder et al. 1973).

- The onset of symptoms following *M. fulvius* envenomation occurs within minutes to hours after the bite (Kitchens and Van Mierop 1987).
- Patients who sustain *M. fulvius* bites may develop ptosis, progressive weakness, hypersalivation, respiratory, and cardiac arrest. (Weiss and McIsaac 1971; Kitchens and Van Mierop 1987).
- *M. tener* bites in the US are associated with more local tissue effects than *M. fulvius* (Fernandez 2009).

How Does Botulism Toxin Produce Neurologic Symptoms?

- Botulinum toxin binds to the cell membrane of cholinergic nerve terminals in the peripheral nervous system. Once bound to the cell membrane, the botulinum toxin enters the nerve terminal through endocytosis and permanently incapacitates proteins in the presynaptic nerve terminal that assist with exocytosis of acetylcholine. The inability to release acetylcholine at peripheral nerve endings leads to weakness and paralysis. (Dressler et al. 2005; Shukla and Sharma 2005)
- Botulinum toxin does not cross blood brain barrier, and thus, does not affect central acteylcholine synapses.
- Ultimately, presynaptic nerve terminals must regenerate for patients to recover.
- Botulinum antitoxin only works on circulating toxin, not toxin that has bound to the presynaptic nerve terminals.

Diagnostic Testing

WBC	Hemoglobin	Platelets
10.8 k/mm^3	12.5 g/dL	205 k/mm^3

Na	K	Cl	CO_2	BUN/Cr	Glucose
139 mmol/L	4.1 mmol/L	109 mmol/L	23 mmol/L	8/0.95 mg/dL	68 mg/dL

INR: 1.1
Fibrinogen: 2.3 g/L
CK: 143,174 IU/L
ABG: pH 7.35, pCO2 50 mmHg, pO2 95 mmHg

Ancillary Testing Performed in an Australian Hospital

Australian Snake Venom detection kit was positive for Death Adder venom.

What Venoms Are Tested for with the Australian Snake Venom Detection Kit, also Called the CSL™ SVDK (CSL 2007)?

- Death adder
- Tiger snake
- Brown snake
- Black snake
- Taipan snake

What Specimens Can Be Used to Test for Venom with the Snake Venom Detection Kit, Which Can Only Be Used for Detecting Australian Snake Envenomations?

- Urine if the patient is already experiencing systemic toxicity
- The bite site itself, even if washed
- A swab from fangs of a dead snake

Hospital Course

As antivenin was being drawn up, within 1 h of the envenomation, the patient deteriorated with respiratory arrest and bradycardia. He was intubated without any medications and mechanically ventilated. He was hemodynamically stable, but profoundly paralyzed. Neurological exam revealed flaccid paralysis with unreactive pupils.

There Are Two Types of Antivenin (AV) Available in Australia for Death Adder Envenomations, Polyvalent and Monovalent. What Is the Difference Between the Two Types of Antivenin?

Monovalent AV, of which there are five types of snake AV, contains at least one type of Australian snake AV. Polyvalent AV contains all five types of AV, and hence, has the largest volume of AV per vial (Isbister et al. 2013). There is also a separate AV for sea snake.

Why Is Monovalent Antivenin a Better Choice for Treatment of a Known Death Adder Envenomation?

Polyvalent AV has a higher risk of anaphylactoid reactions due to its larger volume of foreign protein. Therefore, monovalent AV is preferable in clinical scenarios where envenomation can be narrowed down to a single snake group (Isbister et al. 2013).

When Should Antivenin (AV) Be Given in Death Adder Envenomations? What Is the Recommended Dose?

- AV should be commenced as soon as there are signs of ptosis and bulbar palsy with a positive VDK result.
- If there is a definitive identification of the snake and signs of ptosis or bulbar palsy but no VDK available, give AV.
- Negative inspiratory force (NIF) measurements can be followed to detect impending respiratory failure/worsening respiratory muscle involvement
- Current practice is to give only 1 vial AV and repeat the dose if symptoms are progressing (Isbister et al. 2013)

Hospital Course Continued

By the end of the antivenin infusion, the patient was able to move his left fingers and within 15 min his entire left arm. Overnight, he could subsequently wiggle his toes, lift his left arm, and obey some commands. Neostigmine was given as a bolus and infusion on hospital day two. The patient had improved respiratory effort and was extubated on hospital day four. Ultimately, he was discharged home on hospital day eight.

Why Would Neostigmine Be Considered for Use in This Patient?

Neostigmine is a peripheral cholinesterase inhibitor, thus promoting acetylcholine transmission at neuromuscular junctions. Much as it is used in postoperative recovery for reversal of muscle paralysis, it has been tried in death adder envenomation. There are mixed reports of improvement in neurotoxic symptoms related to death adder envenomation in patients receiving neostigmine (Currie et al. 1988; Flachsenberger and Mirtschin 1994; Johnston et al. 2012; Lalloo et al. 1996; Little and Pereira 2000).

Where Do the Toxins in Death Adder Venom from Australasia Act?

Both pre- and post-synaptic neurotoxins are found in the venom of death adders. These cause rapid profound muscular paralysis in systemic envenomation (Wickramaratna and Hodgson 2001).

What Does a Death Adder Look Like? What Features Distinguish It from Other Venomous Snakes in Australasia?

Death adders are elapid snakes with two upper fangs and powerful jaw muscles. They look different to other venomous snakes in Australia due to their short fat bodies, usually under 50 cm length, and diamond-shaped heads. The other distinguishing feature is their short wisp-like tail, which they use to attract prey.

What Are the Indications for Pressure Immobilization Bandage (PIB)? How Does One Apply It on a Bitten Patient? What Are the Potential Pros and Cons of PIB?

In Australia, the pressure bandage and immobilization technique are indicated for all snake bites, including sea snakes. Theoretically, the PIB reduces lymphatic flow of venom and provides time to reach medical care in a bitten patient. PIB is also indicated in funnel-web spider bite, blue-ringed octopus sting, and cone snail sting.

It is applied by using a crepe or elastic bandage to wrap the entire bitten limb, e.g., toes to groin or fingertips to axilla. Immobilization of the limb with a splint and keeping the patient still are also important aspects of preventing venom circulation. The PIB is not intended to act as a vascular tourniquet and care should be taken to prevent reduced blood flow to the bandaged limb.

PIB are not indicated in the management of native North American snakebites (O'Connor et al. 2011).

What Are Some of the Acute and Longer-Term Adverse Effects of Snake Antivenin Administration?

Acute (minutes to hours): anaphylaxis or anaphylactoid reactions to foreign protein. Anaphylaxis is an IgE-mediated event that requires previous sensitization/exposure to antivenin, drug, or protein. Anaphylactoid reactions are difficult to differentiate from anaphylactic reactions as the symptoms are identical. However, anaphylactoid reactions are not mediated by IgE and occur without previous exposure to the antivenin, drug, or protein. Anaphylactoid reactions are often related to the rate of infusion when they occur with antidote administration. In both cases, antivenin administration should be halted and patients should receive a β-agonist, antihistamine, and corticosteroid. With anaphylaxis, if antivenin is needed, patients may need to be on concomitant epinephrine infusion. With anaphylactoid reactions, the infusion can be restarted at a slower rate with careful observation and frequent reassessment of the patient for signs of recurrent anaphylactoid symptoms (Pizon et al. 2011).

Sub-acute (days to weeks): serum sickness. Serum sickness is a delayed immunological response that occurs 7–10 days after exposure to antivenin or drug. Typical symptoms include myalgias, fever, rash, and joint pain. Treatment includes antihistamines and a 2–3 week steroid taper (Pizon et al. 2011).

Case Conclusion

In this case, the patient was bitten and envenomated by a death adder. He required intubation and supportive care for the neurotoxic effects of the venom, in addition to antivenin. As the Australian Snake Venom kit tested positive for death adder venom, he was given monovalent death adder antivenin with improvement in neurologic symptoms. Ultimately, he recovered and was discharged after 8 days of hospitalization.

Specialty-Specific Guidance

Internal Medicine/Family Medicine

- Pressure immobilization bandages may be applied at the time of envenomation to help prevent systemic circulation of venom. These are only beneficial for certain types of envenomations outside the US.
- Onset of neurologic symptoms can be delayed up to 18–24 h after death adder envenomation.
- If you are treating a patient with a possible death adder envenomation, you should contact your local poison control center immediately for treatment guidance and assistance in identifying from where specific antivenin can be obtained.
- AV should be commenced as soon as there are signs of ptosis and bulbar palsy with a positively identified snake or, if you have access to it, a positive VDK result.
- If there is a definitive identification of the snake and signs of ptosis or bulbar palsy but no VDK available, give AV.
- When AV is required, it is preferred to give monovalent AV to limit volume infused and risk for allergic reaction.
- Negative inspiratory force (NIF) measurements can be followed to detect impending respiratory failure/worsening respiratory muscle involvement.

- Current practice is to give only 1 vial AV and repeat the dose if symptoms are progressing.
- AV should be administered under the direction of a medical toxicologist, when available.

Emergency Medicine

- Pressure immobilization bandages may be applied at the time of envenomation to help prevent systemic circulation of venom. These are only beneficial for certain types of envenomations.
- Onset of neurologic symptoms can be delayed up to 18–24 h after death adder envenomation.
- If you are treating a patient with a possible death adder envenomation, you should contact your local poison control center immediately for treatment guidance and assistance in identifying from where specific antivenin can be obtained.
- AV should be commenced as soon as there are signs of ptosis and bulbar palsy with a positively identified snake or, if you have access to it, a positive VDK result.
- If there is a definitive identification of the snake and signs of ptosis or bulbar palsy but no VDK available, give AV.
- When AV is required, it is preferred to give monovalent AV to limit volume infused and risk for allergic reaction.
- Negative inspiratory force (NIF) measurements can be followed to detect impending respiratory failure/worsening respiratory muscle involvement.
- Current practice is to give only 1 vial AV and repeat the dose if symptoms are progressing.
- AV should be administered under the direction of a medical toxicologist, when available.

Toxicology

- Pressure immobilization bandages may be applied at the time of envenomation to help prevent systemic circulation of venom. These are only beneficial for certain types of envenomations.
- Onset of neurologic symptoms can be delayed up to 18–24 h after death adder envenomation.
- AV should be commenced as soon as there are signs of ptosis and bulbar palsy with a positively identified snake or, if you have access to it, a positive VDK result.
- If there is a definitive identification of the snake and signs of ptosis or bulbar palsy but no VDK available, give AV.
- When AV is required, it is preferred to give monovalent AV to limit volume infused and risk for allergic reaction.

- Negative inspiratory force (NIF) measurements can be followed to detect impending respiratory failure/worsening respiratory muscle involvement.
- Current practice is to give only 1 vial AV and repeat the dose if symptoms are progressing.

Neurology

- Onset of neurologic symptoms can be delayed up to 18–24 h after death adder envenomation.
- Negative inspiratory force (NIF) measurements can be followed to detect impending respiratory failure/worsening respiratory muscle involvement.

References

CSL Snake Venom Detection Kit Product Leaflet. 2007. http://www.csl.com.au/docs/92/398/SVDK_Product_Leaflet,0.pdf. Accessed 30 Dec 2015.

Currie B, Fitzmaurice M, Oakley J. Resolution of neurotoxicity with anticholinesterase therapy in death adder envenomation. Med J Aust. 1988;148(10):522–5.

Dressler D, Saberi F, Barbosa E. Botulinum toxin. Arq Neuropsiquiatr. 2005;63(1):180–5.

Fernandez MC. Clinical and demographic aspects of coral snake envenomations in Texas. J Med Toxicol. 2009;5(4):251.

Flachsenberger W, Mirtschin P. Anticholinesterases as antidotes to envenomation of rats by the death adder (Acanthophis antarcticus). Toxicon. 1994;32(1):35–9.

Isbister G, Brown S, Page C, McCoubrie D, Greene S, Buckley N. Snakebite in Australia: a practical approach to diagnosis and treatment. Med J Aust. 2013;199:763–8.

Johnston CI, et al. Death adder envenoming causes neurotoxicity not reversed by Antivenom—Australian Snakebite Project (ASP-16). PLoS Negl Trop Dis. 2012;6(9):e1841.

Kitchens C, Van Mierop L. Envenomation by the eastern coral snake (*Mircrurus fulvius fulvius*): a study of 39 victims. JAMA. 1987;258(12):1615–8.

Lalloo DG, et al. Neurotoxicity, anticoagulant activity and evidence of rhabdomyolysis in patients bitten by death adders (Acanthophis sp.) in southern Papua New Guinea. Q J Med. 1996;89:25–35.

Little M, Pereira P. Successful treatment of presumed death-adder neurotoxicity using anticholinesterases. Emerg Med. 2000;12:241–5.

Norris R, Pfalzgraf R, Laing G. Death following coral snake bite in the United States – First documented case (with ELISA confirmation of envenomation) in over 40 years. Toxicon. 2009;53:693–7.

O'Connor A, Ruha A, Levine M. Pressure immobilization bandages not indicated in the prehospital management of North American snakebites. J Med Toxicol. 2011;7(3):251.

Pizon A, Riley B, Ruha AM. Antivenom (Crotaline). In: Nelson LS, et al., editors. Goldfrank's Toxicologic Emergencies. 9th ed. New York: McGraw-Hill; 2011. p. 1613.

Shukla H, Sharma S. Clostridium: botulinum: a bug with beauty and weapon. Crit Rev Microbiol. 2005;31(1):11–8.

Snyder G, Ramsey H, Taylor W, Chiou C. Neuromuscular blockade of chick biventer cervicis nerve muscle preparation by a fraction from coral snake venom. Toxicon. 1973;11:505–8.

Weiss R, McIsaac R. Cardiovascular and muscular effects of venom from coral snake, Micrurus fulvius. Toxicon. 1971;9:219–28.

Wickramaratna JC, Hodgson WC. A pharmacological examination of venoms from three species of death adder (Acanthophis antarcticus, Acanthophis praelongus and Acanthophis pyrrhus). Toxicon. 2001;39:209–16.

Case 6
Medication Error in the Delivery Room

1. What is given in the delivery room to cause the problem?
2. What is the pathophysiology?
3. How should this neonate be treated?
4. What is the long-term prognosis?
5. How can this medical error be avoided?

Abstract Neonatal medication errors occur in the delivery room, particularly when maternal medications are given in the same location by the same personnel. Ergot derivatives, given to control maternal postpartum hemorrhage, may cause seizures and vasoconstriction in the newborn. Treatment is directed at supportive management to reverse these effects. Other medications which may be involved in a delivery room error are discussed.

Keywords Ergotism • Medication errors • Infant • Newborn • Postpartum hemorrhage

Case: A 1-day-old female becomes hypoxic in the delivery room

History of Present Illness

A full-term, 2.75 kg girl is born after a normal gestation, via uncomplicated vaginal delivery. Apgar scores are 9 and 9. Standard medications are administered to the infant in the delivery room, after which she becomes flushed and cries. Shortly thereafter, her oxygen saturation falls to 85% on room air.

L.R. Dye et al. (eds.), *Case Studies in Medical Toxicology*,
DOI 10.1007/978-3-319-56449-4_6

Physical Examination

Blood pressure	Heart rate	Respiratory rate	O_2 saturation
60/40 mmHg	166 bpm	35 breaths/min	94% on 2 L NC

General: Newborn infant, crying
HEENT: Pupils dilated, sluggishly reactive to light, perioral cyanosis
Cardiovascular: Regular rate and rhythm, no murmurs
Pulmonary: Clear to auscultation, symmetric breath sounds
Abdominal: Soft, non-tender, normal bowel sounds
Neurologic: Global hypotonia
Skin: Warm and well perfused; w/o excessive dryness or diaphoresis

About 1 h later, her oxygen saturation falls to 74%, and she develops shallow respirations. A medication error is suspected and the poison control center is contacted. Naloxone 0.1 mg/kg IV is administered with improvement in tone though no improvement in oxygenation. CPAP with 30% oxygen is applied, and the patient is admitted to the NICU where she develops oliguria and recurrent tonic seizure activity.

What Is Given in the Delivery Room?

The delivery room and perinatal period can be intense and hectic with multiple patients receiving treatment. These factors make this situation very prone to medication errors (Fariello and Paul 2005). Medications available in the delivery room include analgesics, anti-infectives, corticosteroids, antihypertensives, antiepileptics, uterotonics, and tocolytics, in addition to medications used in adult and neonatal resuscitation (Briggs and Wan 2006a; Briggs and Wan 2006b). Of these, fetal respiratory depression can result from magnesium sulfate and opioid analgesics and vasopressin may result in diffuse vasoconstriction. Any of these medications could have caused some of the symptoms initially seen in the neonate described in this case.

Uterotonics are used both in the induction of labor as well as the prophylaxis and treatment of postpartum hemorrhage and include oxytocin, prostaglandins, and ergot derivatives. Two ergots have been used, methylergonovine and ergometrine. Methylergonovine, typically administered intramuscularly, is recommended as the second-line uterotonic (after uterine massage and oxytocin) due to decreased postpartum hemorrhage-related morbidity, when compared to carboprost (Butwick et al. 2015). Ergometrine can also be administered intramuscularly and has been recommended as an adjunct to oxytocin for postpartum hemorrhage following caesarian section (Lourens and Paterson-Brown 2007). Additionally, ergometrine,

Table 1 Obstetric medications used in the delivery room

Agent	Mechanism of action	Therapeutic use	Adverse effects in neonate
Opioid analgesics	Bind opioid receptors to alleviate pain	Treatment of pain, IV or epidural use	Respiratory and CNS depression
Magnesium sulfate	Smooth muscle relaxant	Treatment of pre-eclampsia and eclampsia	Respiratory and CNS depression
Vasopressin	Vasoconstriction	Treatment of hypotension	Vasoconstriction, seizures
Uterotonics: Oxytocin Methylergonovine Ergometrine	Vasoconstriction, smooth muscle contraction	Prevention of postpartum hemorrhage, treatment of uterine atony	Vasoconstriction, seizures, respiratory failure, oliguria

combined with oxytocin, can be given intramuscularly and will cause decreased morbidity compared to oxytocin alone, but has higher rates of hypertension and stroke. Both ergots may also be administered orally and intravenously, but have greater variability in clinical effects and higher rates of adverse effects (Gizzo et al. 2013) (Table 1).

Shortly after administration, the delivery room staff discovered that the patient was given methylergonovine 0.2 mg IM, intended for the mother to reduce uterine bleeding. It was confused for vitamin K by the delivery room nurse. It appears that the syringes of vitamin K and methylergonovine were prefilled and stored nearby each other. It is unclear how the error was discovered, but the baby developed symptoms rather quickly and the poison control center was contacted from the delivery room.

What Is the Pathophysiology of Neonatal Ergotism?

The uterotonics cause vasoconstriction and smooth muscle contraction and are used to prevent postpartum hemorrhage and uterine atony. However, when given to a newborn infant, vasoconstriction is the dominant feature. Seizures, respiratory failure progressing to arrest, and oliguria are reported (Donatini et al. 1993; Aeby et al. 2003).

How Should Neonatal Ergot Poisoning Be Treated?

Treatment is focused on inducing vasodilation and enhancing circulation. Nitroprusside has been effective in several case reports but other agents have been employed (Bangh et al. 2005). Intravenous fluids will increase urine output. Anticonvulsants may be needed, as in this case. Additionally, there may be a benefit to naloxone. There is 60–70% structural similarity between methylergonovine and morphine suggesting that reversal of respiratory depression caused by the ergot may be due to naloxone's antagonism at opioid receptors (Sullivan et al. 2013).

NICU Course

In the NICU, the patient was endotracheally intubated and treated with phenobarbital and magnesium for seizures. There was improvement in hypertension and seizures ceased. In addition to maintenance fluids, boluses of D10W were administered for oliguria with a resultant increase in urine output.

On the second day of life, the patient was evaluated with an EEG, showing no further seizure activity. A head ultrasound demonstrates no intracranial hemorrhage, and magnetic resonance imaging revealed no ischemic injuries. The patient was discharged home on hospital day 7 without focal neurological deficits and no apparent long-term sequelae.

What Is the Long-Term Prognosis After Neonatal Ergot Poisoning?

The long-term effects of the seizures and respiratory depression due to neonatal ergot toxicity are not well described. Neonatal mortality is noted in 6% of reported cases though these deaths occurred over 30 years ago and advances in neonatal intensive care may have improved more recent outcomes (Bangh et al. 2005).

How Can This Medical Error Be Avoided?

The cause of the patient's symptoms in this case is a well-described medication error: the confusion between a syringe containing a uterotonic, such as methylergonovine or oxytocin, intended for the mother, and vitamin K, intended for the neonate. While this specific error has been described for over 40 years, reports actually increased in the 1990s (Bangh et al. 2005).

Preventing medical errors is a major challenge to healthcare providers. In neonates, dosing errors are the most common, with tenfold dosing errors making up a significant proportion of these (Connors et al. 2014). Although controlled studies have not been performed, strategies which may reduce the risk of mistaking an ergot for vitamin K include delaying the administration of vitamin K until the baby is transferred to the newborn nursery, utilizing two nurses, one solely responsible for administering medication to the mother and another responsible for treating the neonate, and color coding medications or syringes to denote those meant for the mother or child (Bangh et al. 2005).

Specialty-Specific Guidance

Neonatology/Obstetrics

- In the neonate who develops unexpected decompensation after medication administration in the delivery room, consider a medication error.
- If respiratory depression is the predominant feature, consider opioid analgesics or magnesium sulfate.
- In the neonate with seizures and respiratory depression, consider neonatal ergotism from inadvertent administration of a uterotonic.

Toxicology

- Neonatal ergot poisoning is primarily characterized by hypertension and seizures, the consequence of uncontrolled vasoconstriction.
- Treatment options include:
  - Management of hypertension with vasodilating agents
  - Anticonvulsant therapy
  - IV fluids to enhance urine output and improve perfusion
  - Naloxone, due to structural similarity of methylergonovine with morphine

References

Aeby A, Johansson AB, De Schuiteneer B, Blum D. Methylergometrine poisoning in children: review of 34 cases. J Toxicol Clin Toxicol. 2003;41:249–53.

Bangh SA, Hughes KA, Roberts DJ, Kovarik SM. Neonatal ergot poisoning: a persistent iatrogenic illness. Am J Perinatol. 2005;22:239–43.

Briggs GG, Wan SR. Drug therapy during labor and delivery, part 1. Am J Health Syst Pharm. 2006a;63:1038–47.

Briggs GG, Wan SR. Drug therapy during labor and delivery, part 2. Am J Health Syst Pharm. 2006b;63:1131–9.

Butwick AJ, Carvalho B, Blumenfeld YJ, El-Sayed YY, Nelson LM, Bateman BT. Second-line uterotonics and the risk of hemorrhage-related morbidity. Am J Obstet Gynecol. 2015;212(5):642.e1–7.

Connors NJ, Nelson LS, Hoffman RS, Su MK. Neonatal medication errors reported to a poison control center. Clin Tox. 2014;52:326. (abstract).

Donatini B, Le Blaye I, Krupp P. Inadvertent administration of uterotonics to neonates. Lancet. 1993;341:839–40.

Fariello JY, Paul E. Patient safety issues in a tertiary care hospital's labor and delivery unit. AWHONN Lifelines. 2005;9:321–3.

Gizzo S, Patrelli TS, Gangi SD, Carrozzini M, Saccardi C, Zambon A, Bertocco A, Fagherazzi S, D'antona D, Nardelli GB. Which uterotonic is better to prevent the postpartum hemorrhage? Latest news in terms of clinical efficacy, side effects, and contraindications: a systematic review. Reprod Sci. 2013;20:1011–9.

Lourens R, Paterson-Brown S. Ergometrine given during caesarean section and incidence of delayed postpartum haemorrhage due to uterine atony. J Obstet Gynaecol. 2007;27:795–7.

Sullivan R, Nelsen J, Duggineni S, Holland M. Management of methylergonovine induced respiratory depression in a newborn with naloxone. Clin Toxicol (Phila). 2013;51:47–9.

Case 7
Delirium and Bradycardia Following Opioid Dependency Treatment

1. What are the suspected agent and its action?
2. Describe the pharmacokinetics of this agent.
3. What are contraindications to the use of this agent?
4. What are other complications seen with this agent?
5. How does naltrexone differ from naloxone?
6. How common is delirium with opioid withdrawal? How does precipitated opioid withdrawal differ from withdrawal due to abstinence?
7. What are other treatment options for a patient experiencing acute withdrawal following an injection of this agent?
8. What other agents are approved by the FDA for the management of the opioid dependence?

Abstract This case involves a 69-year-old male who presented to the emergency department from the primary care provider with acute delirium and agitation following the administration of a medication to treat opioid dependency. The patient was agitated and moved all extremities purposefully, but did not follow any commands. He was given benzodiazepines, but ultimately required intubation. He made a complete recovery. This case discusses various medications and regimens to treat opioid withdrawal. In addition, this case discusses treatment options for patients with acute pain who are concurrently taking medications to facilitate abstinence.

Keywords Delirium • Opioid detoxification • Vivitrol® • Delirium • Opioid dependence

L.R. Dye et al. (eds.), *Case Studies in Medical Toxicology*,
DOI 10.1007/978-3-319-56449-4_7

History of Present Illness

A 69-year-old male is transported to the Emergency Department (ED) by ambulance from a primary care clinic with acute delirium, agitation, vomiting, and incontinence. The symptoms began very shortly after the administration of an intramuscular medication used to treat opioid dependency. Prior to this injection, the patient was reportedly normal. During transport, the patient receives 2 mg intramuscular naloxone, 4 mg intramuscular ondansetron, and 0.3 mg of subcutaneous epinephrine without any change in his clinical status.

Past Medical History	Hypertension, chronic kidney disease, anxiety, depression, chronic pain syndrome, and substance abuse
Medications	Metoprolol, amlodipine, furosemide, duloxetine, and pantoprazole
Allergies	No known drug allergies

Physical Examination

Blood pressure	Heart rate	Respiratory rate	Temperature	O_2 saturation
154/73 mmHg	110–130 bpm	24 breaths/min	37.4 °C (99.32 °F)	99% (room air)

General: Agitated, diaphoretic, and was thrashing in the gurney.
HEENT: Pupils were mid-size and briskly reactive.
Neck: Supple without meningeal findings.
Cardiovascular: Tachycardia rhythm.
Pulmonary: Lungs clear bilaterally.
Neurologic: The patient exhibited purposeful movements of all extremities but did not follow any commands. No clonus or rigidity.

Initial Treatment

A capillary glucose was obtained and was determined to be 199 mg/dL. Intravenous access was established and the patient received a total of 40 mg of intravenous diazepam over 20 min without any improvement in delirium or agitation. Ultimately, the patient required endotracheal intubation and escalating doses of propofol. He was ultimately admitted to the intensive care unit, on a continuous infusion of propofol at 50 ug/kg/min.

A call to the physician's office revealed the patient had received an intramuscular injection of Vivitrol®.

Diagnostic Testing

Na	K	Cl	CO_2	BUN	Cr	Glucose
143 mmol/L	3.3 mmol/L	102 mmol/L	25 mmol/L	27 mg/dL	2.0 mg/dL	180 mg/dL

Creatine kinase: 89 IU/L.
Serum ethanol, salicylate, and ethanol levels all non-detectable.

Ancillary Testing

CT head: negative for hemorrhage or masses.
An EKG revealed sinus tachycardia with normal intervals and no ischemic changes. Urine toxicology screen (immunoassay; Siemens EMIT) revealed the presence of opiates, phencyclidine, and tetrahydrocannabinol (THC). Amphetamines, barbiturates, benzodiazepines, and cocaine were not detected.

Case Continuation

In the ICU, he was maintained on propofol 50–60 mcg/kg/min overnight. He was tachycardic to 90–120 bpm and hypertensive with a mean arterial pressure between 90 and 120 mm Hg, despite propofol. His hypertension was treated with labetalol. After 18 h, the propofol infusion was tapered, and he was extubated without difficulty 23 h following his initial presentation.

His hospital course was relatively uneventful after that. He was transitioned to his oral anti-hypertensives with improved blood pressure control. He received a total of 8 mg lorazepam over the next 7 days, mostly at night for insomnia and anxiety. He reported that he had recently been using methadone purchased from a friend to treat chronic pain. He was evaluated by psychiatry and refused counseling or any rehabilitation services.

What Is Vivitrol®?

Vivitrol® is a sustained release microsphere formulation of naltrexone administered by deep intramuscular (IM) injection every 4 weeks. Naltrexone is a potent competitive opioid receptor antagonist with a five to sevenfold greater affinity for mu receptors than naloxone. It also exhibits greater affinity at delta and kappa receptors (Toll et al. 1998). Vivitrol® incorporates naltrexone into microspheres of a polylactide-co-glycolide polymer that slowly releases a dose of 380 mg naltrexone over weeks as the polymer is degraded. It received FDA approval for the treatment of alcohol dependence in 2006 and for the treatment of opioid dependence in 2010.

Naltrexone is also available for oral administration as 50 mg tablets (Revia®).

Describe the Pharmacokinetics of Naltrexone?

After oral administration naltrexone undergoes extensive first pass metabolism to 6-β-naltrexol. 6-β-naltrexol, an active metabolite, is cleared more slowly than naltrexone. After oral dosing, the apparent serum half-lives of naltrexone and 6-β-naltrexol are about 10 and 11 h respectively although a very prolonged terminal elimination phase for naltrexone of 96 h has been measured in adults (Verebey et al. 1976). With chronic dosing serum 6-β-naltrexol levels exceed those of naltrexone, more so following oral administration. Although 6-β-naltrexol is a less potent antagonist and does not access the CNS as rapidly as naltrexone, 6-β-naltrexol likely contributes to the long duration of central opioid antagonism seen with naltrexone (Yancey-Wrona et al. 2009; Porter et al. 2002). Both naltrexone and 6-β-naltrexol undergo glucuronidation and renal elimination.

After intramuscular administration of Vivitrol®, there is an early serum peak of naltrexone within hours followed by a second peak about 2 days later. After that there is sustained plateau concentration of naltrexone for several weeks followed by a slow decline. Naltrexone concentrations over 2 ng/mL are maintained for nearly 5 weeks after injection of 380 mg Vivitrol®. The elimination half-life of naltrexone administered as Vivitrol® is about 5 days, with the terminal elimination of naltrexone dependent on the degradation of the microsphere polymer (Dunbar et al. 2006; Bigelow et al. 2012).

What Are Contraindications to the Use of Vivitrol®?

Contraindications to the use of this product include current opioid dependence or withdrawal. Because of the risk of precipitated withdrawal the manufacturer recommends patients be opioid free for 7–10 days, and up to 2 weeks following use of methadone or buprenorphine. An intramuscular or intranasal naloxone challenge can be considered.

An approach used by one addiction specialist prior to administration of Vivitrol® is to first confirm the absence of opioids in urine (opiates, methadone, buprenorphine) and then administer a test dose of 0.1 mg naloxone intranasal (IN). If there is no reaction to this, an increased dose of 1 mg naloxone IN is administered. If the patient exhibits no withdrawal symptoms to this second dose, then Vivitrol® is administered.

What Are Other Complications Seen with Vivitrol®?

Other complications of Vivitrol® include local reactions at the injection site and depressed mood. The risk of opioid overdose following escalating doses of an opioid in an attempt to overcome naltrexone's opioid antagonism is also a concern, as is heightened opioid sensitivity after discontinuation of Vivitrol® (Product Insert 2014).

How Does Naltrexone Differ from Naloxone?

Naltrexone has a higher affinity for mu opioid receptors compared to naloxone, along with a longer half-life and a longer duration of action. Both naltrexone and naloxone undergo hepatic first pass metabolism. Although naltrexone undergoes extensive first pass hepatic metabolism the dose used orally for abstinence treatment, 50 mg, is sufficient to allow adequate systemic bioavailability. Additionally, naltrexone has an active metabolite, 6-β-naltrexol.

How Common Is Delirium with Opioid Withdrawal? How Does Precipitated Opioid Withdrawal Differ from Withdrawal Due to Abstinence?

The typical features of withdrawal from abstinence include malaise, anxiety, restlessness, insomnia, yawning, lacrimation, rhinorrhea, sweating, nausea, vomiting, myalgia, cramps, diarrhea, and piloerection. Alertness is typically preserved and delirium is not a usual feature.

Opioid antagonist precipitated withdrawal can present more dramatically and include agitation and delirium, as seen in this case. Other symptoms reported include posturing, incontinence, confusion, delusions, and hallucinations (Quigley and Boyce 2001; Singh et al. 2009; Boyce et al. 2003; Mannelli et al. 1999; Sheeram et al. 2001). In a small series of patients using naltrexone as part of rapid opioid detoxification nearly 25% of patients exhibited delirium (Golden and Sakhrani 2004). Other complications of rapid opioid detoxification include pulmonary edema, seizures, protracted vomiting with dehydration, esophageal tear, and mediastinitis (Hamilton et al. 2002).

What Are Other Treatment Options for a Patient Experiencing Acute Withdrawal Following an Injection of Vivitrol®?

Treatment of a patient experiencing withdrawal after injection of Vivitrol® is challenging. Previous cases that involved implantation of a naltrexone pellet afforded the option of surgical removal of the implant (Hamilton et al. 2002). As a depot given by deep IM injection, this option would be a more difficult undertaking and likely pose a greater risk of complications.

There is limited experience describing the use of the partial mu agonist buprenorphine to treat precipitated withdrawal after oral naltrexone. A 44-year-old woman with acute opioid withdrawal after a 50 mg oral dose of naltrexone had relief of her withdrawal symptoms 45 min after a 4 mg sublingual dose of buprenorphine (Santos and Hernandez 2013). Buprenorphine has also been used in the outpatient setting to attenuate opioid withdrawal in methadone-dependent patients undergoing accelerated opioid detoxification with naltrexone (Urban and Sullivan 2008).

The use of GABAergic agents such as benzodiazepines can be used to achieve sedation in the acutely agitated, delirious patient from opioid withdrawal. Anti-emetics can be used to manage uncontrolled nausea.

Clonidine, an alpha-2 agonist, ameliorates symptoms associated with opioid withdrawal. Opioid withdrawal is associated with noradrenergic hyperactivity in several areas of the brain, including the locus coeruleus and caudal medulla neurons projecting to the bed nucleus of the stria terminalis. Stimulation of presynaptic alpha-2 receptors in these regions reduces noradrenergic output by these neurons (Aghajanian 1978; Delfs et al. 2000). Dexmedetomidine, a short-acting parenteral centrally active alpha-2 agonist is a lesser studied alternative if enteral administration of clonidine is not possible.

In this case, sedation was treated, first with a benzodiazepine and then, after observing no effect with 40 mg diazepam, proceeding with escalating doses of propofol until adequate sedation was achieved.

What Other Agents Are Approved by the FDA for the Management of the Opioid Dependence?

Besides abstinence-based programs, management of the opioid-dependent person may involve substitution treatment with methadone or buprenorphine.

Opioid substitution therapy has been a traditional approach to opioid addiction going back over a century. Methadone has been the standard opioid used as replacement therapy since the 1960s. First synthesized in Germany in the 1930s, studies at Rockefeller University in the 1960s demonstrated efficacy in the management of opioid addiction. Methadone has a long duration of action, allowing once daily or even less frequent dosing for treatment of dependency. At larger doses, it blocks the reinforcing euphoria from parenterally used opioids (Green et al. 2004). A reduction in the illicit use of opioids, a reduction in criminal behavior and incarceration, reduced rates of infectious complications from intravenous drug abuse and reduced mortality are all attributed to methadone maintenance therapy (Farrell et al. 1994). Some detoxification programs use a tapering dose of methadone over days to weeks, with abstinence the goal at the completion of detoxification.

Buprenorphine is a potent, partial mu agonist. It possesses a high affinity for the mu receptor but without full agonist activity. A ceiling analgesic effect is observed and a bell-shaped dose response curve suggests antagonist effects at higher doses (Orman and Gillian 2009; Johnson et al. 2003). A highly lipophilic drug, buprenorphine has a plasma elimination half-life of about 3–5 h, but because of its very high affinity and slow dissociation from mu receptors its duration of action is prolonged, with a terminal elimination half-life of over 24 h (National Institute on Drug Abuse 1992). Buprenorphine can block the effects of other pure opioid agonists, displacing full opioid agonists from the mu receptor and precipitating withdrawal (Orman and Gillian 2009; National Institute on Drug Abuse 1992; Lewis 1985). Because of this risk buprenorphine should always be initiated in a supervised medical setting.

Specialty-Specific Guidance

Internal Medicine/Family Medicine

- In addition to absence programs, pharmacologic treatment options to facilitate opioid dependence include naltrexone, methadone, and buprenorphine.
- Patients need to be opioid free for at least 7–10 days (or 2 weeks in the case of prior methadone or buprenorphine administration) prior to starting Vivitrol®.

Prehospital

- While patients in opiate withdrawal may be agitated, true delirium is very uncommon.
- Naloxone should not be administered in the absence of features consistent with opiate toxicity (e.g., bradypnea), as its administration may precipitate withdrawal.

Emergency Medicine

- The emergency physician may encounter difficulty adequately treating pain during an acute painful condition in a patient on an opiate antagonist.
- While simultaneously searching for alternative etiologies of delirium, the emergency physician should promptly administer benzodiazepines.
- Advanced airway management, including endotracheal intubation may be required for patients with refractory agitation.

Addiction Medicine

- It is imperative to ensure that the patient has no evidence of opiates remaining in the system prior to administering a long-acting narcotic analgesic.
- Some experts recommend a test dose of naloxone prior to administering Vivitrol®.

References

Aghajanian GK. Tolerance of locus coeruleus neurones to morphine and suppression of withdrawal response by clonidine. Nature. 1978;276:186–8.

Bigelow GE, Preston KL, et al. Opioid challenge evaluation of blockade by extended-release naltrexone in opioid-abusing adults: dose-effects and time-course. Drug Alcohol Depend. 2012;123:57–65.

Boyce SH, Armstrong PAR, et al. Effect of inappropriate naltrexone use in a heroin misuser. Emerg Med J. 2003;20:381–2.

Delfs JM, Zhu Y, et al. Noradrenaline in the ventral forebrain is critical for opiate withdrawal-induced aversion. Nature. 2000;403:430–4.

Dunbar JL, Turncliff RZ, et al. Single- and multiple-dose pharmacokinetics of long-acting injectable naltrexone. Alcohol Clin Exp Res. 2006;30:480–90.

Farrell M, Ward J, et al. Fortnightly review: methadone maintenance treatment in opioid dependence: a review. BMJ. 1994;309:997.

Golden SA, Sakhrani DL. Unexpected delirium during rapid opioid detoxification (ROD). J Addictive Diseases. 2004;23:65–75.

Green M, Kellogg S, Kreek MJ. Methadone: history, pharmacology, neurobiology, and use. In: Adelman G, Smith B, editors. Encyclopedia of neuroscience. 3rd ed. Amsterdam: Elsevier; 2004.

Hamilton RJ, Olmedo RE, et al. Complications of ultrarapid opioid detoxification with subcutaneous naltrexone pellets. Acad Emerg Med. 2002;9:63–8.

Johnson RE, Strain EC, et al. Buprenorphine: how to use it right. Drug Alcohol Depend. 2003;70:S59–77.

Lewis JW. Buprenorphine. Drug Alcohol Depend. 1985;14:363–72.

Mannelli P, DeRisio S, et al. Serendipitous rapid detoxification from opiates: the importance of time-dependent processes. Addiction. 1999;94:589–91.

National Institute on Drug Abuse. Buprenorphine: an alternative treatment for opioid dependence. Research Monograph 121, U.S. Dept. Health and Human Services; 1992.

Orman JS, Gillian MK. Buprenorphine/naloxone. A review of its use in the treatment of opioid dependence. Adis Drug Evaluation. 2009;69:577–607.

Porter SJ, Somogyi AA, et al. In vivo and in vitro potency studies of 6 beta-naltrexol, the major human metabolite of naltrexone. Addict Biol. 2002;7:219–25.

Product Insert. Vivitrol. Alkermes, Inc. Waltham, MA. Accessed 22 Dec 2014.

Quigley MA, Boyce SH. Unintentional rapid opioid detoxification. Emerg Med J. 2001;18:494–5.

Santos C, Hernandez SH. A case of unintentional naltrexone induced opioid withdrawal successfully treated with buprenorphine in an emergency department setting (abstract). Clin Toxicol. 2013:332–3.

Sheeram SS, McDonald T, et al. Psychosis after ultrarapid opiate detoxification (letter). Am J Psychiatry. 2001;158:970.

Singh SM, Sharma B, et al. Unintentional rapid opioid detoxification: case report. Psychiatr Danub. 2009;21:65–7.

Toll L, Berzetei-Gurske IP, et al. Standard binding and functional assays related to medications development division testing for potential cocaine and opiate narcotic treatment medications. NIDA Res Monogr. 1998;178:440–66.

Urban V, Sullivan R. Buprenorphine rescue from naltrexone-induced opioid withdrawal during relatively rapid detoxification from high-dose methadone: a novel approach. Psychiatry (Edgmont). 2008;5(4):56–8.

Verebey KV, Volavka J, et al. Naltrexone: disposition, metabolism, and effects after acute and chronic dosing. Clin Pharmacol Ther. 1976;20:315–28.

Yancey-Wrona JE, Raymond TJ, et al. 6-Beta-naltrexol preferentially antagonizes opioid effects on gastrointetinal transit compared to antinociception in mice. Life Sci. 2009;85:413–20.

Case 8
Necrotic Skin Lesion

1. What is the differential diagnosis for a necrotic skin ulcer?
2. What is the difference between a bite and a sting?
3. What is the habitat of this spider?
4. What is the composition of the venom of this spider?
5. How is the diagnosis made?
6. Describe the different clinical presentations of envenomation by this spider.
7. What laboratory testing is should be obtained in suspected envenomation from this spider?
8. What is the optimal management?
9. How can one avoid getting bitten by this spider?

Abstract A 41-year-old female presented to the emergency department with a lesion on her left forearm. The patient suspected she was bitten 3 days prior by something while cleaning her attic. She subsequently developed a fever (103 °F), chills and myalgias throughout the course of the day. This chapter reviews possible causes of this patient's symptomatology, including a thorough discussion of spider envenomation with focus on *Loxosceles reclusa*, commonly known as the brown recluse spider.

Keywords Loxoscelism • Loxosceles • Loxosceles reclusa • Brown recluse • Necrotic arachnidism • Spider envenomation

L.R. Dye et al. (eds.), *Case Studies in Medical Toxicology*,
DOI 10.1007/978-3-319-56449-4_8

History of Present Illness

Day 1

A 41-year-old female was moving from a new home and, while she was cleaning the attic, she developed a burning pain in the left forearm. She was concerned that she may have spilled a cleaning fluid on her arm, but also noticed several spiders in the area. She took a shower and applied aloe, but developed itching at the site that lasted all night.

Day 2

The patient woke up with a blister on her left forearm and noted a "bull's eye" appearance. The area swelled progressively through the course of the day. She applied baking soda and meat tenderizer to the site without relief.

Day 3

By the third morning, the blister progressed to a severely pruritic, enlarged necrotic, pale lesion within an erythematous ring demarcating the lesion. She developed a fever and myalgia as the day progressed. She went to the emergency department (ED) .

Past Medical History	None
Medications	Daily multivitamin Denies herbals and OTC drugs
Allergies	Penicillin (rash)
Social History	Denies tobacco, ethanol or other drugs of abuse. Lives with her husband (a chemistry professor) and 2 children, ages 8 and 13 years old. She works part-time as a graphic designer

Physical Examination

Blood pressure	Heart rate	Respiratory rate	Temperature	O_2 saturation
110/70 mmHg	110 bpm	17 breaths/min	39.4 °C (102.92 °F)	100% (room air)

General: Vital signs stable, febrile, and in mild distress
HEENT: Pupils equal and reactive. No congestion or rhinorrhea
Cardiovascular: Tachycardia but regular rhythm
Pulmonary: Chest clear to auscultation bilaterally without wheezes, rales, or rhonchi.
Abdomen: Soft, non-tender
Neurologic: Alert and oriented, normal cognition, no tremor

Skin: Indolent necrotic appearing lesion enclosed within an irregular, erythematous ring of ecchymosis on left forearm

EKG showed sinus tachycardia.

ED Course

Over a 6 h stay in the ED, the patient's fever resolved with ibuprofen. Her vitals remained stable throughout her ED stay. She received a tetanus booster, wound debridement, and a wound culture was obtained. She was instructed to alternate between acetaminophen and ibuprofen for any pain. A diagnosis of suspected spider bite was made, and she was discharged with instructions to follow up with her primary medical doctor (PMD) in a couple of days.

Day 5

She went to her PMD for follow-up. The necrotic lesion had enlarged since her ED visit. She was prescribed cephalexin and instructed to use triple antibiotic ointment along with topical corticosteroids as needed. The fever resolved, but she had persistent myalgia.

Day 30

The patient went to her PMD for a second follow-up. She completed the course of antibiotics and topical treatments. The wound ulceration was increased since her last visit but was noted to be healing. She had no complaints of pain or any systemic symptoms. She was no longer using topical treatments on the wound.

Year 1

The patient had a permanent scar on left forearm at the site of the necrotic lesion.

What Is the Differential Diagnosis for a Necrotic Skin Ulcer?

- Diabetic ulcer
- Anthrax
- Chemical corrosive burns
- Viral skin infection (chronic herpes simplex)

- Bacterial skin infection (community-acquired methicillin-resistant Staphylococcus aureus MRSA)
- Fungal skin infection
- Steven–Johnsons syndrome
- Lyme disease
- Localized vasculitis
- Necrotic fasciitis
- Toxicodendron dermatitis (poison ivy, poison oak)
- Squamous cell carcinoma
- Erythema multiforme
- Brown recluse spider bite
- Syphilitic chancre
- Kissing bug (Triatoma genus) bites

What Is the Difference Between a Bite and a Sting?

Arachnids can bite or sting. A bite is defined as the creation of a wound using the oral pole with the intention of envenomation, whereas a sting occurs from an ovipositor at the aboral pole (also able to function in egg laying) (Hahn 2011). Spiders inflict bites. Nearly all spiders are venomous, but very few spiders are capable of envenomating humans because they cannot penetrate the skin.

Spider Facts

Many humans fear spiders evoking the term Arachnophobia. In reality, spiders rarely bite humans, but when they do, it is usually as a means of self-defense. Of the more than 41,000 species of spiders worldwide, there are an estimated 100 species of loxosceles (Isbister and Fan 2011), and most of them live in S. America. In the United States, there are thought to be about 12 species of loxosceles. The *Loxosceles reclusa*, also known by the common name brown recluse, is the most prevalent spider, found predominantly in South-Central and the Midwest US. (Wilson et al. 2005). It is most active during the spring to fall months, and hibernates otherwise. The brown recluse spider's venom has been found to contain both cytotoxic and hemotoxic properties.

Characteristics of a Brown Recluse Spider

The brown recluse spider when fully grown is about the size of a US quarter including the legs (Wilson et al. 2005). It is described as yellow, gray, orange, or brown in color ranging in size from 6–20 mm (Hahn 2011). Contrary to other spider species with eight eyes, the brown recluse has three pairs of eyes (dyads), one in front and two pairs on the side of its cephalothorax, arranged in a semicircle formation (Andersen et al. 2011).

The brown recluse has a large leg to body ratio (~5:1), and the female is relatively larger and more dangerous compared to the male. They are heat tolerant, forming uneven, small, flocculent, adhesive webs for laying eggs or sleeping (Rhoads 2007). The brown recluse has a brownish violin-shaped ("fiddle back spider") mark on its dorsum of the cephalothorax. It has a life span of approximately 2 years and is a nocturnal hunter, preferring warm, dark, dry places. They are typically nonaggressive, preferring quiet environments (hence the name recluse), but will bite when threatened. Most bites are reported at nighttime, but early morning bites occur more commonly in the summer months. They are purported to be capable of surviving up to 6 months without a food source or water and can tolerate extremes in temperature (Hahn 2011).

What Is the Habitat of a Brown Recluse Spider?

Brown recluse spiders are nocturnal foragers, with flat bodies, that facilitate their ease of adaptation to their environment. They are most commonly found in dark places where they can easily hide such as rocks or basements.

What Is the Composition of Brown Recluse Venom?

The amount of venom imparted with each bite will vary, with some bites delivering up to 0.5 cc (Rhoads 2007). The venom of the brown recluse spider is composed of many different enzymes—the most problematic constituents of the venom include **sphingomyelinase-D** (necrosis) and **hyaluronidase** (spreading factor) although other subcomponents, including deoxyribonuclease, ribonuclease, esterase, proteases, collagenase, alkaline phosphatase, and lipase contribute to morbidity (Hahn 2011). Collectively, the venom constituents have cytotoxic and hemotoxic properties.

Mechanism of destruction: Once envenomed, sphingomyelinase-D causes red blood cell hemolysis and causes the platelets to release serotonin (Hahn 2011). Next, hyaluronidase functions as a spreading factor, facilitating further penetration of venom and destruction. The downstream release of inflammatory mediators leads to vessel thrombosis, low platelet counts, ischemia of the tissue, and renal failure (Rhoads 2007). Coagulation and vascular occlusion ultimately lead to a necrotic ulcer (Hahn 2011).

How Is the Diagnosis Made?

The only definitive way to identify a brown recluse bite is to have it identified by an entomologist or arachnologist although it is often unavailable. There is presently no lab test to confirm a suspected brown recluse spider bite. Several techniques have been used in research (but none are useful in clinical practice):

- Lymphocyte transformation test (measures lymphocytes that have undergone blast transformation up to 1 month post envenomation) (Hahn 2011).
- Passive hemagglutination inhibition test in guinea pigs (venom inhibits antiserum-induced agglutination of venom-coated erythrocytes) (Hahn 2011).
- Enzyme-linked immunoassay(ELISA) in rabbits (Found to confirm venom up to 4 days post envenomation, and antigen up to 21 days post envenomation) (Hahn 2011).

Describe the Different Clinical Presentations of Loxosceles Envenomation

The clinical manifestations of a brown recluse spider bites are divided into three categories (Hahn 2011):

- Cutaneous loxoscelism
  When a minute amount of venom is delivered, skin destruction is minimal to absent. The initial reaction often consists of erythema, pain, and/or pruritus. A small vesicle may form at the area of the bite, and the vesicle develops into a lesion that takes on a "bull's eye" appearance—a central vesicle surrounded by blanching enveloped by an erythematous, ecchymotic area (can be delayed in onset-hours to days). When the vesicle ruptures, it exposes an ulcer. The size of the ulcer and amount of venom will determine the time of healing.
- Necrotic arachnidism
  In severe envenomation, necrosis of the blister can occur 3–4 days post envenomation, with eschar formation between 5 and 7 days. In 7–14 days, the wound becomes indurated and the eschar can slough. The ulceration heals by secondary wound closure (Hahn 2011). Local necrosis tends to be more severe over fatty areas (Hahn 2011). Large lesions can take weeks or months to heal and leave permanent scars.
- Systemic loxoscelism
  Systemic effects develop rarely in 24–48 h after envenomation. Mild effects include fever, chills, myalgias, arthralgias, and generalized rash. Severe systemic effects occur rarely and may include hemolysis, jaundice, renal failure, and shock (Hahn 2011).

What Laboratory Testing Is Obtained in Suspected Brown Recluse Envenomation?

- Complete blood count (CBC), PT/INR.
- Markers for hemolytic anemia (haptoglobin).
- Creatine phosphokinase to detect rhabdomyolysis.
- Potassium should be obtained in patients with hemolysis.
- Renal function to screen for renal insufficiency.

Any suspected brown recluse spider bite warrants careful scrutiny of the extent of skin integrity and destruction. It is important to note that systemic reactions are related to the degree of envenomation and is not predictive of the cutaneous reaction. Fatalities from brown recluse spider bites have been reported and most have occurred in children <7 years of age from subsequent massive hemolysis (Rhoads 2007). Fatalities from renal failure secondary to hemoglobinuria, leukocytosis, thrombocytopenia, and disseminated intravascular coagulation have also been reported (Rhoads 2007).

What Is the Optimal Management?

Management of necrotic arachnidism is controversial, but the mainstay is proper wound care, tetanus prophylaxis, analgesia/antipruritic as needed. Slow wound healing is classically observed with severe brown recluse envenomation; therefore, continued follow-up to monitor the progression of symptomatology and providing supportive care is prudent. Multiple treatment modalities have been tried and are discussed below, but it is important to note that **the efficacy has not been proven and many are controversial**.

- Analgesia—used supportively and symptomatically
- Antipruritic—commonly used
- Cold packs (purported to decrease venom enzymatic activity and pain), avoid heat (may spread venom activity)
- Dapsone in early studies found to inhibit local infiltration of the wound by polymorphonuclear leukocytes, but carries the risk of potential methemoglobinemia (particularly in G6PD patients), hemolysis, or hepatitis
  - Now is generally avoided (Hahn 2011)
- Hyperbaric oxygen therapy (promotes angiogenesis, but results are not conclusive and not recommended) (Andersen et al. 2011)
- Steroids may decrease red cell destruction, but also healing (Mold and Thompson 2004) and should be avoided
- Antibiotics—useful for secondary infections
- Antivenom—South American countries—Brazil, Peru, Mexico, and Argentina may use horse-derived F(ab) which may reduce cutaneous and prevent systemic loxoscelism. Usually not used if >72 h have passed since envenomation. Brazil has two antivenoms available from the Brazilian ministry of health: antiloxoscelic serum and anti-arachnidic serum.
- Surgical debridement—early surgery (first 2 months post bite) may cause inflammation and potentially worsen the chances of healing and is usually avoided (Andersen et al. 2011).

(Hahn 2011; Wright et al. 1997; Mold and Thompson 2004; Micromedex 2016)

How Can One Avoid Getting Bitten by a Brown Recluse Spider?

Preventing contact with a brown recluse spider via chemical control pesticides, insect repellants, and wearing long sleeves is the best way to avoid envenomation. Most brown recluse spider bite envenomation cases resolve largely without incident.

Case Conclusion

In this case, the patient presented with evidence of necrotic arachnidism. Her symptoms were managed with tetanus prophylaxis, wound care, analgesia, and an empiric course of oral antibiotic. Her wound culture resulted negative. Many conditions may mimic brown recluse spider bites and many tried treatments have shown little promise and are largely controversial. Improper diagnosis may lead to amputation, acute renal failure, and death.

Specialty-Specific Guidance

Internal Medicine/Family Medicine

- Many spiders bite, and many are brown, but most of those bites are unlikely to be a brown recluse spider bite.
- Prevention of brown recluse spider bites in at-risk populations (disabled elderly, crawling children) is important.
- The use of safe and effective pesticides and insect repellants should be encouraged during at-risk months in South-central and Midwest US.
- Educating patients to wear long sleeves while outdoors is important during active brown recluse spider months.
- Thorough follow-up is imperative for any suspected spider bite to monitor for progression of symptoms.
- Discussion of the potential for slow healing and proper wound care should be communicated to the patient or caregiver.

Pediatrics

- Crawling and inquisitive infants are at risk for spider bites.
- The pediatric population has been found to be most at risk for fatalities in the literature.

- Caregivers need to be vigilant with proper wound care measures in the home setting.
- Discuss the need for proper and safe insect control in at-risk social settings.

Emergency Medicine

- It is important to note that alleged spider bites may in reality be infections, especially community-acquired methicillin-resistant Staphylococcus aureus (MRSA).
- There is currently no available antivenom in the United States for brown recluse spider bites.
- The mainstay of treatment is supportive and symptomatic care, including tetanus prophylaxis and proper wound care.
- Recognize that patients may return with worsening symptoms since brown recluse spider bites may worsen before improving.
- Encourage follow-up with the PMD for monitoring progression of symptoms over weeks/months.

Toxicology

- Annually, a number of spider bites are reported to the 55 poison control centers nationwide. Most of these bites tend to be fairly innocuous.
- There is no effective antidote in the United States for *Loxosceles reclusa* spider bites.
- Obtain a thorough history of the exposure to rule out other causes of symptomatology.
- There is no specific lab or test that can definitively diagnose a brown recluse bite.

Nephrology

- Acute renal failure is a rare but grave consequence of brown recluse spider bites.
- In addition, rhabdomyolysis and hemoglobinuria have been reported.
- Thorough monitoring of renal labs and supportive care is important in cases of systemic loxoscelism

Infectious Disease

- Patients who are initially diagnosed as having community-acquired MRSA may instead have been bitten by a brown recluse spider bite.

- Note that *clostridium perfringens* have been cultured from the fangs and venom of the brown recluse spider and may lead to secondary infection (Mold and Thompson 2004).
- Secondary infection is uncommon even with extensive necrotic lesions.

References

Andersen RJ, Campoli J, Johar SK, Schumacher KA, Jr JA, E. Suspected brown recluse envenomation: a case report and review of differential treatment modalities. J Emerg Med. 2011;41(2):e31–7.

Hahn I. Arthropods. In: Nelson LS, Lewis NA, Howland MA, Hoffman RS, Goldfrank LR, Flomenbaum NE, editors. Goldfrank's Toxicologic Emergencies. 9th ed. New York: McGraw-Hill; 2011. p. 1564–7.

Isbister GK, Fan HW. Spider bite. Lancet. 2011;378:2039–47.

Micromedex. Brown recluse spider bites. Accessed Apr 3 2016.

Mold JW, Thompson DM. Management of brown recluse spider bites in primary care. JABFP. 2004;17(5):347–52.

Rhoads J. Epidemiology of the brown recluse spider bite. J Am Acad Nurse Pract. 2007;19:79–85.

Wilson JR, Hagood CO, Prather ID. Brown recluse spider bites: a complex problem wound. A brief review and case study. Ostomy Wound Management. 2005;51(3):59–66.

Wright SW, Wrenn KD, Murray L, Seger D. Clinical presentation and outcome of brown recluse spider bite. Ann Emerg Med. 1997;30(1):28–32.

Case 9
Isoniazid Ingestion

1. What are the typical characteristics of seizures associated with isoniazid overdose?
2. Was the dose of isoniazid in this case sufficient to cause a seizure?
3. What is the mechanism by which isoniazid overdose causes seizures?
4. What is pyridoxine's mechanism as an antidote in isoniazid poisoning?
5. How is pyridoxine dosed when treating isoniazid overdose?
6. Is oral pyridoxine equivalent to intravenous pyridoxine for seizure prophylaxis in isoniazid poisoning?
7. What is the mechanism of lactic acidosis associated with isoniazid toxicity?
8. What general treatment should be initiated?
9. What other treatment(s) may be helpful?
10. What are the other toxic effects of isoniazid?
11. Has toxicity ever been associated with pyridoxine administration?

Abstract Isoniazid is commonly used in treatment of latent *Mycobacterium tuberculosis* infections. We report a case of a 6-year-old boy that had a seizure following an accidental overdose of isoniazid. The pathophysiology, clinical manifestations, evaluation, and treatment of isoniazid toxicity are discussed. The mechanism of action and use of pyridoxine (Vitamin B_6) as an antidote to isoniazid and hydrazine poisoning is reviewed.

Keywords Isoniazid • Pyridoxine • Hydrazine • Tuberculosis • Overdose • Status epilepticus

L.R. Dye et al. (eds.), *Case Studies in Medical Toxicology*,
DOI 10.1007/978-3-319-56449-4_9

History of Present Illness

A 6-year-old boy inadvertently received an extra dose of his own isoniazid. He had been on the medication for about 1 week for treatment of latent tuberculosis and the error occurred due to a miscommunication between his parents. Each parent had given the boy his usual daily isoniazid dose, about 2 h apart. The total amount of isoniazid received was 450 mg. The regional poison center was contacted and calculated the dose he received as 38 mg/kg. They recommended immediate evaluation at the nearest emergency department. The child was brought to the emergency department by his parents and appeared well with no symptoms at the time of his initial evaluation.

Past Medical History	Microcephaly Cerebral Palsy No prior history of seizure disorder Latent tuberculosis
Medications	Isoniazid
Allergies	NKDA
Family History	Adopted, unknown
Social History	Lives with both adoptive parents

Physical Examination

Blood pressure	Heart rate	Respiratory rate	Temperature	O2 saturation
130/70 mmHg	104 bpm	24 breaths/min	37 °C (98.6 °F)	98% (room air)

General: Well appearing, under-developed for age

HEENT: Normocephalic, atraumatic, and extraocular movements intact; pupils are equal, round, and reactive to light

Cardiovascular: Regular rate and rhythm, normal S1 and S2. Extremities are warm and well perfused

Pulmonary: Unlabored respirations, symmetric chest expansion, clear breath sounds

Abdominal: Bowel sounds normal. Soft, non-tender, and nondistended

Neurologic: Alert, oriented, mild cognitive delay for age (at baseline), normal reflexes, normal tone, and no focal deficits

Diagnostic Testing

WBC	Hemoglobin	Hematocrit	Platelets	Differential
10 k/mcL	13.5 gm/dL	35%	200 k/mm^3	N/A

Na	K	Cl	CO_2	BUN	Cr	Glucose
138 mEq/L	4.2 mEq/L	102 mEq/L	25 mEq/L	18 mg/dL	0.7 mg/dL	110 mg/dL

AST: 28 U/L (reference range: <42 U/L)
ALT: 6 U/L (reference range: <35 U/L)

The consulting toxicologist recommended the child be admitted to the hospital overnight for observation.

Hospital Course, Day One

The poison center recommended prophylactic pyridoxine administration. The treating hospital did not have intravenous pyridoxine available, so 450 mg of oral pyridoxine was administered approximately 3 h after the isoniazid ingestion.

Seven hours after the ingestion, the child had normal vital signs and no symptoms. Nine hours after the ingestion, the boy had a single, generalized, tonic-clonic seizure that lasted several seconds. He was given 1 mg of lorazepam and the convulsive activity stopped. Following the episode, the child was drowsy but returned to baseline mental status within 30 min following the incident. Neurology was consulted. There were no focal deficits on neurologic exam. No further pyridoxine or benzodiazepines were administered. There were no further seizure-like episodes and the patient was not placed on prophylactic anticonvulsants.

What Are the Typical Characteristics of Seizures Associated with Isoniazid Overdose?

Seizures may occur as early as 30 min following isoniazid overdose and are expected to be refractory to conventional antiepileptic drugs (Whitefield and Klein 1971). In patients who remain asymptomatic during observation in the emergency department, seizures or other signs of acute toxicity are unlikely to occur more than 6 h after acute isoniazid ingestion or overdose.

Was the Dose of Isoniazid in This Case Sufficient to Cause a Seizure?

Seizures may occur at isoniazid doses greater than 20 mg/kg. Doses greater than 35 mg/kg are very likely to cause seizures, as in this case, where an estimated 38 mg/kg was ingested (Alvarez and Guntupalli 1995). Seizures associated with therapeutic doses of isoniazid have been very rarely reported (Tsubouchi et al. 2014).

What Is the Mechanism by Which Isoniazid Overdose Causes Seizures?

Ultimately, isoniazid (INH) leads to depletion of the inhibitory neurotransmitter γ-aminobutyric acid (GABA). The subsequent lack of inhibitory neurotransmission allows seizures to occur unchecked. Isoniazid leads to GABA depletion by altering the metabolism of pyridoxine (Vitamin B_6), a coenzyme in a number of key biotransformation reactions (Biehl and Vilter 1954). Isoniazid metabolites cause a functional pyridoxine deficiency by inhibiting pyridoxine phosphokinase, an enzyme responsible for converting pyridoxine to its active form, pyridoxal-5′-phosphate (PLP). In addition, active pyridoxine is complexed with isoniazid metabolites and renally excreted, depleting pyridoxine levels. Finally, isoniazid inhibits glutamic acid decarboxylase (GAD), which catalyzes the synthesis of GABA from glutamate. The combined relative excess of glutamate and GABA deficiency leads to the seizures for which isoniazid is well known (Fig. 1). Hydrazine and methylated hydrazines, as found in rocket fuels and *Gyromitra esculenta* (False morel) mushrooms cause seizures by a similar mechanism (Leathem and Dorran 2007).

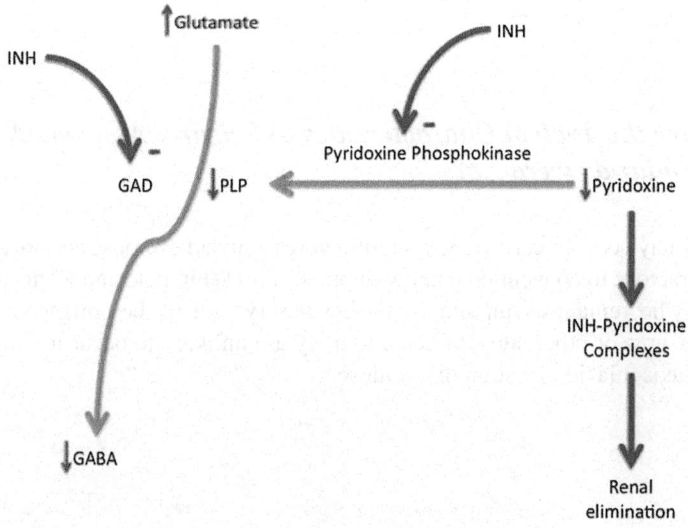

Fig. 1 Isoniazid effects on pyridoxine metabolism and GABA synthesis

What Is Pyridoxine's Mechanism as an Antidote in Isoniazid Poisoning?

Pyridoxine has been demonstrated to terminate seizures and reverse persistent coma in isoniazid poisoning (Brent et al. 1990; Brown et al. 1984; Wason et al. 1981). Replacing pyridoxine permits catalysis of the conversion of glutamate to GABA, increasing inhibitory neurotransmission. Of note, in addition to the rare genetic disorder pyridoxine-dependent epilepsy, a retrospective review of adults hospitalized with status epilepticus found pyridoxine deficiency in 94%, compared to 39.4% in outpatient historical controls (Dave et al. 2015). Therefore, termination of seizures in response to pyridoxine administration should not be considered diagnostic of isoniazid toxicity.

How Is Pyridoxine Dosed When Treating Isoniazid Overdose?

It is recommended that asymptomatic patients who have ingested potentially toxic amounts of isoniazid within 2 h of presentation receive prophylactic pyridoxine administration. This is based on the time to peak concentration of isoniazid, which is less than 2 h under varied conditions (Peloquin et al. 1999). Dosing of pyridoxine for prophylactic and antidotal use is identical. If the dose of isoniazid is known, the dose of pyridoxine should be equal to the dose of isoniazid ingested on a gram-per-gram basis (Wason et al. 1981). If the dose is unknown, empiric dosing of 5 g of intravenous pyridoxine for adults and 70 mg/kg up to a maximum of 5 g for children has been recommended, infused at 0.5 g/min until seizures terminate or the maximum dose has been given (Lheureux et al. 2005). A volunteer study of intravenous pyridoxine pharmacokinetics demonstrated a short plasma elimination half-life of 0.12 h (Zempleni and Kubler 1994). Some sources have suggested administering any remainder of the pyridoxine dose after seizure termination over 4–6 h (Lheureux et al. 2005) or giving total doses over 4 g as serial 1 g intramuscular injections (APP Pharmaceuticals 2008).

Is Oral Pyridoxine Equivalent to Intravenous Pyridoxine for Seizure Prophylaxis in Isoniazid Poisoning?

There are no published data comparing the use of oral versus intravenous pyridoxine in acute isoniazid poisoning. The oral bioavailability of pyridoxine is estimated at 60–80%, so it is reasonable to consider giving additional pyridoxine or simply doubling the dose if oral pyridoxine must be used (Tarr et al. 1981; Zempleni 1995). Intravenous pyridoxine is preferred due to the lower risk of airway complications/aspiration, should seizure occur, but is not readily available at all facilities.

What Is the Mechanism of Lactic Acidosis Associated with Isoniazid Toxicity?

The classic triad of acute isoniazid poisoning consists of seizures, coma, and severe metabolic acidosis (Watkins et al. 1990). Metabolic acidosis associated with isoniazid toxicity is usually high anion-gap metabolic acidosis with elevated lactate. In animal models of isoniazid poisoning, administration of a neuromuscular blocking agent prevented the development of metabolic acidosis, suggesting that it results from convulsive activity, and is not a drug effect independent from seizures (Chin et al. 1978).

What General Treatment Should Be Initiated?

While preparing and administering antidotal treatment with pyridoxine, airway management should be undertaken as clinically indicated and supportive management of seizures should be provided to prevent secondary injuries. Activated charcoal has been demonstrated to bind isoniazid and prevent absorption when given *immediately* following ingestion (Siefkin et al. 1987). However, when given 1 h after experimental ingestion there was no significant reduction in the area under the concentration-time curve or the half-life of isoniazid (Scolding et al. 1986). Early (less than 1 h post-ingestion) administration of activated charcoal should therefore be weighed carefully against the risk of aspiration and seizure.

What Other Treatment(s) May Be Helpful?

Benzodiazepines may be ineffective alone until GABA is replenished (Campo-Soria et al. 2006) but have synergistic antiepileptic effects when given with pyridoxine (Chin et al. 1978). Barbiturates and other GABA-agonists would be expected to have similar synergistic effects. Current evidence-based guidelines for the treatment of status epilepticus do not address the use of pyridoxine (Glauser et al. 2016). However, because conventional antiepileptics without GABA-agonism, such as phenytoin, are ineffective in treating isoniazid toxicity and most other drug-induced seizures, empiric administration of pyridoxine in known or suspected isoniazid poisoning has been recommended (Wills and Erickson 2005; Chen et al. 2016).

A study of chronic hemodialysis patients suggested minimal recovery (median = 9%) of an isoniazid dose in dialysate (Malone et al. 1999). A recent pharmacokinetic analysis of one overdose case treated with continuous venovenous hemodiafiltration (CVVHDF) suggested significant isoniazid clearance was possible with hemodialysis if started as early as possible (Skinner et al. 2015). Given the rapid elimination of isoniazid and that most patients can be treated with benzodiazepines and pyridoxine, more human evidence is needed before the use of hemodialysis can be recommended.

Hospital Course, Day Two

The child was seen by the neurology service. It remained unclear whether or not isoniazid toxicity was primarily responsible for the seizure in this case. It was suspected that his outpatient dose was based on confusion of his weight in kilograms for a weight in pounds, since he was unusually small for his age. Given the child's underlying cerebral palsy and chronic illness, it was postulated that he may have an underlying predisposition to seizures but it was difficult to attribute the seizure to a new epileptiform disorder given the temporal association with isoniazid administration. The child was scheduled for neurology follow-up and an electroencephalogram (EEG). He had no further seizures and was discharged to home in stable condition on hospital day two.

What Are the Other Toxic Effects of Isoniazid?

Isoniazid-induced coma is reported in severe acute poisoning and may be prolonged up to 72 h (Brown et al. 1984). The exact mechanism of coma is unknown, but its reversal has been reported with repeated doses of pyridoxine (Brent et al. 1990).

In chronic use, the most common adverse effect of isoniazid therapy is peripheral neuropathy, typically in a stocking-glove distribution. It is recommended that patients at high risk of developing isoniazid-induced peripheral neuropathy, such as those with HIV infection, malnutrition, alcoholism, and diabetes, receive pyridoxine supplementation with isoniazid therapy (Cilliers et al. 2010; van der Watt et al. 2011). Isoniazid is also associated with both idiopathic autoimmune hepatitis and direct hepatocellular injury and has resulted in hepatic failure when the drug was continued after development of transaminase elevation (Goldman and Braman 1972). Though animal models demonstrate that hepatic steatosis can be prevented by concomitant pyridoxine administration (Whitehouse et al. 1983), there is no human evidence supporting its use to reverse isoniazid-induced hepatotoxicity. Current understanding of isoniazid-induced hepatic injury does not suggest a mechanism for pyridoxine as an antidote (Hassan et al. 2016).

Has Toxicity Ever Been Associated with Pyridoxine Administration?

Though pyridoxine has a wide therapeutic window, it is neurotoxic in chronic and acute overdose. Small and large fiber ataxic neuropathy has occurred in chronic overuse of pyridoxine supplementation (Cohen and Bendich 1986). Inadvertent overdose of antidotal pyridoxine has also been reported, with two patients, each of whom received greater than 2 g/kg of parenteral pyridoxine over a 3-day period, developing severe sensory neuropathy and persistent inability to ambulate 1 year after the event (Albin et al. 1987).

Specialty-Specific Guidance

Internal Medicine/Family Medicine

- Isoniazid may cause peripheral neuropathy and hepatitis in chronic use.
- Pyridoxine supplementation is recommended for patients taking isoniazid at high risk for developing neuropathy.
- Fulminant liver failure may result if unrecognized.
- Acute isoniazid poisoning results in neurotoxicity (seizures, coma) due to GABA depletion.
- Pyridoxine is antidotal for isoniazid neurotoxicity but does not treat hepatotoxicity.
- Accidental ingestions by children may be potentially toxic and merit emergency department observation and prophylactic pyridoxine administration.
- When in doubt, obtain medical toxicology consultation (In the United States, 1-800-222-1222).

Emergency Medicine

- Seizures due to isoniazid toxicity result from GABA depletion and are refractory to antiepileptics such as phenytoin.
- The antidote for isoniazid neurotoxicity (seizures, coma) is pyridoxine.
- Benzodiazepines may be synergistic with pyridoxine but may not work alone.
- Consider isoniazid toxicity in patients with refractory seizures and supporting or unknown history.
- Pyridoxine is unlikely to cause harm when dosed appropriately and may be considered for refractory seizures or status epilepticus of unknown cause.
- When in doubt, obtain medical toxicology consultation (In the United States, 1-800-222-1222).

Toxicology

- Isoniazid causes both functional and true pyridoxine depletion.
- In the absence of pyridoxal-5′-phosphate (PLP), glutamic acid decarboxylase (GAD) cannot convert glutamate to GABA, resulting in seizures.
- Lactic acidosis secondary to isoniazid overdose appears to result from convulsive activity and may be prevented by neuromuscular blockade.
- Pyridoxine has been demonstrated to reverse both acute seizures and protracted coma resulting from isoniazid ingestion.
- Benzodiazepines may be synergistic with pyridoxine but may not work alone.
- Pyridoxine itself may cause small and large fiber neuropathy in chronic overuse or acute manifold overdose.

References

Albin RL, Albers JW, Greenberg HS, Townsend JB, Lynn RB, Burke JM Jr, Alessi AG. Acute sensory neuropathy-neuronopathy from pyridoxine overdose. Neurology. 1987;37(11):1729–32.
Alvarez FG, Guntupalli KK. Isoniazid overdose: four case reports and review of the literature. Intensive care medicine. 1995;21(8):641–4.
APP Pharmaceuticals, L. Pyridoxine Hydrochloride Injection, USP [package insert]. 2008. http://editor.fresenius-kabi.us/PIs/Pyridoxine_Inj_45817E_Apr_08.pdf. Accessed 30 July 2015.
Biehl JP, Vilter RW. Effects of isoniazid on pyridoxine metabolism. J Am Med Assoc. 1954;156(17):1549–52.
Brent J, Vo N, Kulig K, Rumack BH. Reversal of prolonged isoniazid-induced coma by pyridoxine. Arch Intern Med. 1990;150(8):1751–3.
Brown A, Mallett M, Fiser D, Arnold WC. Acute isoniazid intoxication: reversal of CNS symptoms with large doses of pyridoxine. Pediatr Pharmacol (New York). 1984;4(3):199–202.
Campo-Soria C, Chang Y, Weiss DS. Mechanism of action of benzodiazepines on GABAA receptors. Br J Pharmacol. 2006;148(7):984–90.
Chen HY, Albertson TE, Olson KR. Treatment of drug-induced seizures. Br J Clin Pharmacol. 2016;81(3):412–9.
Chin L, Sievers ML, Laird HE, Herrier RN, Picchioni AL. Evaluation of diazepam and pyridoxine as antidotes to isoniazid intoxication in rats and dogs. Toxicol Appl Pharmacol. 1978;45(3):713–22.
Cilliers K, Labadarios D, Schaaf HS, Willemse M, Maritz JS, Werely CJ, Hussey G, Donald PR. Pyridoxal-5-phosphate plasma concentrations in children receiving tuberculosis chemotherapy including isoniazid. Acta Paediatr. 2010;99(5):705–10.
Cohen M, Bendich A. Safety of pyridoxine--a review of human and animal studies. Toxicol Lett. 1986;34(2–3):129–39.
Dave HN, Eugene Ramsay R, Khan F, Sabharwal V, Irland M. Pyridoxine deficiency in adult patients with status epilepticus. Epilepsy Behav. 2015;52(Pt A):154–8.
Glauser T, Shinnar S, Gloss D, Alldredge B, Arya R, Bainbridge J, Bare M, Bleck T, Dodson WE, Garrity L, Jagoda A, Lowenstein D, Pellock J, Riviello J, Sloan E, Treiman DM. Evidence-based guideline: treatment of convulsive status epilepticus in children and adults: report of the guideline committee of the American Epilepsy Society. Epilepsy Curr. 2016;16(1):48–61.
Goldman AL, Braman SS. Isoniazid: a review with emphasis on adverse effects. Chest. 1972;62(1):71–7.
Hassan HM, Guo HL, Yousef BA, Luyong Z, Zhenzhou J. Hepatotoxicity mechanisms of isoniazid: a mini-review. J Appl Toxicol. 2016;35(12):1427–32.
Leathem AM, Dorran TJ. Poisoning due to raw Gyromitra esculenta (false morels) west of the Rockies. CJEM. 2007;9(2):127–30.
Lheureux P, Penaloza A, Gris M. Pyridoxine in clinical toxicology: a review. Eur J Emerg Med. 2005;12(2):78–85.
Malone RS, Fish DN, Spiegel DM, Childs JM, Peloquin CA. The effect of hemodialysis on isoniazid, rifampin, pyrazinamide, and ethambutol. Am J Respir Crit Care Med. 1999;159(5 Pt 1):1580–4.
Peloquin CA, Namdar R, Dodge AA, Nix DE. Pharmacokinetics of isoniazid under fasting conditions, with food, and with antacids. Int J Tuberc Lung Dis. 1999;3(8):703–10.
Scolding N, Ward MJ, Hutchings A, Routledge PA. Charcoal and isoniazid pharmacokinetics. Hum Toxicol. 1986;5(4):285–6.
Siefkin AD, Albertson TE, Corbett MG. Isoniazid overdose: pharmacokinetics and effects of oral charcoal in treatment. Hum Toxicol. 1987;6(6):497–501.
Skinner K, Saiao A, Mostafa A, Soderstrom J, Medley G, Roberts MS, Isbister GK. Isoniazid poisoning: pharmacokinetics and effect of hemodialysis in a massive ingestion. Hemodial Int. 2015;19(4):E37–40.

Tarr JB, Tamura T, Stokstad EL. Availability of vitamin B6 and pantothenate in an average American diet in man. Am J Clin Nutr. 1981;34(7):1328–37.

Tsubouchi K, Ikematsu Y, Hashisako M, Harada E, Miyagi H, Fujisawa N. Convulsive seizures with a therapeutic dose of isoniazid. Intern Med. 2014;53(3):239–42.

van der Watt JJ, Harrison TB, Benatar M, Heckmann JM. Polyneuropathy, anti-tuberculosis treatment and the role of pyridoxine in the HIV/AIDS era: a systematic review. Int J Tuberc Lung Dis. 2011;15(6):722–8.

Wason S, Lacouture PG, Lovejoy FH Jr. Single high-dose pyridoxine treatment for isoniazid overdose. JAMA. 1981;246(10):1102–4.

Watkins RC, Hambrick EL, Benjamin G, Chavda SN. Isoniazid toxicity presenting as seizures and metabolic acidosis. J Natl Med Assoc. 82(1):57, 62, 64.

Whitefield CL, Klein RG. Isoniazid overdose: report of 40 patients, with a critical analysis of treatment and suggestions for prevention. Am Rev Respir Dis. 1971;103:887.

Whitehouse LW, Tryphonas L, Paul CJ, Solomonraj G, Thomas BH, Wong LT. Isoniazid-induced hepatic steatosis in rabbits: an explanation for susceptibility and its antagonism by pyridoxine hydrochloride. Can J Physiol Pharmacol. 1983;61(5):478–87.

Wills B, Erickson T. Drug- and toxin-associated seizures. Med Clin North Am. 2005;89(6):1297–321.

Zempleni J. Pharmacokinetics of vitamin B6 supplements in humans. J Am Coll Nutr. 1995;14(6):579–86.

Zempleni J, Kubler W. The utilization of intravenously infused pyridoxine in humans. Clin Chim Acta. 1994;229(1–2):27–36.

Case 10
Status Epilepticus Following Recreational Drug Insufflation

1. What is your differential diagnosis?
2. What is this agent?
3. On what receptors does this agent act?
4. Does the patient's report of drug used accurately reflect the active ingredient involved?
5. What are the symptoms of toxicity from this agent?
6. What are the symptoms of serotonin syndrome/toxicity?
7. How does cyproheptadine play a role in the management of serotonin syndrome?
8. What are the symptoms of anticholinergic toxicity?
9. What are the symptoms of stimulant toxicity?
10. What other common drugs of abuse cause seizures?
11. Why are bupropion and pregabalin on the differential?

Abstract A 21-year-old male presented to the emergency department in status epilepticus. He was hyperthermic, tachycardic, and hypertensive with hyperreflexia and clonus. Laboratory workup revealed a metabolic acidosis with associated hyperlactatemia. He was admitted to the intensive care unit where he was sedated, mechanically ventilated, and externally cooled. His hospital course was complicated by an aspiration pneumonia and rhabdomyolysis but he fully recovered.

Keywords 25i • N-BOMe • Serotonin syndrome • Seizures • Designer drugs • Phenylethylamine

L.R. Dye et al. (eds.), *Case Studies in Medical Toxicology*,
DOI 10.1007/978-3-319-56449-4_10

History of Present Illness

A 21-year-old male presented to the Emergency Department (ED) in status epilepticus after insufflating a while at a party. The powder had been purchased online. Emergency Medical Services (EMS) was called to the scene after he began seizing. Bystanders initially reported the patient used only mescaline, LSD, and marijuana. The patient received 10 mg of diazepam and was nasally intubated by EMS.

Past Medical History	Unknown
Medications	Unknown
Allergies	Unknown
Family History	Unknown
Social History	Unknown

Physical Examination

Blood pressure	Heart rate	Respiratory rate	Temperature	O_2 saturation
140/80 mmHg	130 bpm	14 breaths/min (intubated)	38.1 °C (105.0 °F)	100%

General: Patient was intubated and manual ventilated with bag valve mask.
HEENT: Normocephalic and atraumatic. Pupils were equal, round, and reactive to light. Mucus membranes were moist.
Cardiovascular: Cardiac exam was significant for tachycardia but otherwise normal.
Pulmonary: Chest was clear to auscultation bilaterally.
Neurologic: The patient had five beats of clonus bilaterally. There was no rigidity but some diffuse extremity hyperreflexia.
Skin: Sweat was present in the axilla.

What Is Your Differential Diagnosis?

- Serotonin syndrome
- Neuroleptic malignant syndrome
- Anticholinergic toxicity
- Cathinone abuse (bath salts, K2, etc.)
- Synthetic stimulant/drug use (e.g., cocaine, amphetamine)
- Pregabalin insufflation
- Bupropion insufflation
- Synthetic marijuana use (spice, K2, etc.)

Diagnostic Testing

WBC	Hemoglobin	Platelets
14.8 k/mm^3	16.5 g/dL	421 k/mm^3

Na	K	Cl	CO_2	BUN/Cr	Glucose
145 mmol/L	4.0 mmol/L	102 mmol/L	5 mmol/L	20/2.2 mg/dL	85 mg/dL

Acetaminophen: negative
Salicylic acid: negative
Ethanol: negative
Urine drug screen: negative for amphetamine, benzodiazepines, cocaine, methadone, and opiates
CK: 403 U/L
ABG: pH: 6.5/ pCO2 82/ pO2 412
Lactate: 22.6 mmol/L
AST: 25 U/L, ALT: 32 U/L
INR: 1.96, PT: 22 s, PTT: 47.6 s

Ancillary Testing

EKG: NSR rate of 95, QRS 110, QTc 500. No acute ischemic changes.
CXR: lungs clear without pneumothorax or effusion
CT Head: no acute abnormality

Hospital Course

Initially in the ED, the patient had a brief period of bradycardia of 40 beats/min. The bradycardia resolved after he was re-intubated orally and given atropine 0.5 mg intravenously. He continued to have intermittent clinically evident seizures in the ED for which he was given a bolus of 2 mg lorazepam and 4 mg midazolam with subsequent resolution. Ultimately, a propofol infusion was started and he was transferred to the MICU.

In the medical ICU, the patient's clinical course was complicated by a right-sided pneumothorax attributed to barotrauma and a chest tube placed. He also developed an aspiration pneumonia. No further seizures were noted once admitted, but the patient continued to have hyperreflexia and clonus. His acidosis resolved within 4 h of mechanical ventilation and fluid resuscitation, but he remained intubated and sedated for 3 days due to persistent agitation, tachycardia, and hyperthermia with trials of decreased sedation. He received infusions of propofol (50 mg/h) and fentanyl (100 mcg/h), and Lactated Ringers at 300 mL/h while intubated.

An external cooling blanket was applied, but he remained febrile and tachycardic for the first 4 days of admission. His creatinine peaked at 2.3 mg/dL on hospital day 2; creatinine kinase peaked at 64,000 U/L, AST 873 U/L, and ALT 295 U/L on hospital day 3, all of which declined prior to discharge. He was extubated on hospital day 3 and made a full recovery.

Upon extubation, the patient reported he insufflated a substance called "N-BOMB" prior to becoming ill.

What Is N-BOMB?

- N-BOMB and N-BOMe are slang terms that refer to any one of several substituted phenylethylamines. The most commonly identified drugs in this group are 25I-NBOMe, 25C-NOBMe, and 25B-NBOMe (Laskowski 2014a; Papoutsis et al. 2015; Poklis et al. 2014; Poklis et al. 2015; Zuba D and Sekula K 2013a; Zuba et al. 2013b).
- These drugs are modified hallucinogens from a class of drugs called the 2C-X family or considered phenylethylamine derivatives.
- N-BOMB and N-BOMe are often marketed as "legal LSD" or psychedelic phenylethylamines (Laskowski 2014; Suzuki 2014).
- N-BOMB is used in microgram doses as a powder or on blotter paper and has been insufflated, ingested, and injected (Lawn et al. 2014).

On What Receptors Does N-BOMB Act On?

- This group of phenylethylamines was initially developed as radioligands for serotonin receptors. They have a high affinity for 5HT2A, but as different groups are substituted on the drug; there are different receptor affinities. Several analogs exist including: 25B-, 25C, 25D-, 25H-, 25I-. They may also have peripheral alpha agonist properties (Laskowski et al. 2014; Johnson et al. 2014; Tang et al. 2014).
- Symptoms of intoxication share similar traits with stimulant and serotonin toxicity (Forrester 2014; Hill et al. 2013; Rose et al. 2013).
- There have been multiple case reports relating intractable seizure activity and death in conjunction with using N-BOMB (Forrester 2014; Hill et al. 2013; Rose et al. 2013).

What Are the Major Hepatic Cytochrome p450 Enzymes Involved in the Metabolism of N-BOMB?

- CYP3A4
- CYP2D6

- This is important information for providers as patients may develop significant drug reactions if they are on a CYP3A4 inhibitor (ex: protease inhibitors or antibiotics like erythromycin) at the time they take N-BOMB (Nielsen et al. 2017).

Does the Patient's Report of Drug Used Accurately Reflect the Active Ingredient Involved?

- It is difficult without confirmation to identify the specific drug abused, and there are private laboratories that can perform confirmatory testing on the parent compound, urine, and blood/serum.
- Confirmatory testing is expensive but warranted in certain cases, such as differentiating between new onset psychosis and drug effect, for epidemiologic tracking, and in any case of suspected child neglect/abuse.
- Confirmatory testing can be obtained from urine or blood using liquid chromatography with tandem mass spectrometry (LC/MS/MS), but may not detect all analogs and will not return in a timely manner to affect clinical care (Lawn et al. 2014; Poklis et al. 2014a, b; Stellpflug et al. 2014).
- There are several analogs that exist for all the designer drugs including N-BOMB, synthetic cathinones, amphetamines, and synthetic marijuana products. They often are sold under one name and may contain a different derivative or different drug all together. For example, the drug "Molly" is being sold on the Internet. "Molly" has traditionally been coined as a street name for ecstasy but in recent years some of the synthetic cathinones are being sold as "Molly" for reported similar highs as those experienced with ecstasy.

What Are the Symptoms and Clinical Effects of Synthetic Phenylethylamine Toxicity?

- Hyperthermia
- Agitation and confusion
- Hallucinations
- Tachycardia
- Rhabdomyolysis
- Seizures
- Excited delirium states
- Serotonin toxicity
- Acute kidney injury
- Metabolic acidosis
- Leukocytosis
- Death

What Are the Symptoms of Serotonin Syndrome/Toxicity?

- Autonomic instability (tachycardia, hypertension, hyperthermia)
- Altered mental status (agitation, delirium)
- Neuromuscular findings (hyperreflexia, clonus, tremor, increased muscle tone)
- Diaphoresis and diarrhea have also been reported

How Does Cyproheptadine Play a Role in the Management of Serotonin Syndrome?

- Cyproheptadine has been used in the treatment of serotonin syndrome because of its 5HT (serotonin) receptor antagonism.
- It is believed cyproheptadine counteracts the effects of serotonin excess by blocking the serotonin receptor.
- While the literature describes some success controlling symptoms of serotonin syndrome, cyproheptadine is an adjunctive therapy to other supportive measures such as benzodiazepines, cooling, and hydration.

What Are the Symptoms of Anticholinergic Toxicity?

- Delirium
- Dry skin (notable in groin and axilla) and dry mucous membranes
- Mydriasis
- Urinary retention
- Hyperthermia
- Flushed and warm skin
- Tachycardia
- Decreased gut motility
- Seizures

What Are the Symptoms of Stimulant Toxicity?

- Tachycardia
- Hypertension
- Mydriasis
- Diaphoresis
- Agitation
- Seizures
- Hyperthermia
- Diarrhea

What Other Common Drugs of Abuse Cause Seizures?

- Cathinones ("bath salts")
- Synthetic marijuana (K2, spice)
- Amphetamines (methamphetamines, ecstasy)
- Cocaine
- Alcohol withdrawal
- Benzodiazepine or barbiturate withdrawal
- Opiates/opioids (respiratory depression can lead to hypoxia and seziures related to hypoxia)
- Phencyclidine

Why Are Bupropion and Pregabalin on the Differential?

- Bupropion is a substituted cathinone that is structurally similar to other phenylethylamines or "bath salts" like mephedrone.
- Bupropion use is associated with decreasing the seizure threshold (Davidson 1989).
- Seizures and QRS prolongation have been reported with both accidental and intentional overdose of buproprion (Curry et al. 2005; Kim and Steinhart 2010; Storrow 1994).
- There are reports of buproprion insufflation as a means of getting high resulting in seizures (Hill et al. 2007; Kim and Steinhart 2010).
- Pregabalin has also been insufflated in effort to get high and has been reported to cause seizures in overdose—both insufflation and ingestion (Reedy 2010; Reedy and Schwartz 2010; Gorodetsky et al. 2012; Schifano et al. 2011).
- There is a case report suggesting AV block after large pregabalin overdose (Aksakal et al. 2012).

Case Conclusion

In this case, a 21-year-old male used a synthetic drug called N-BOMB at a party and developed status epilepticus. The care team provided aggressive supportive care such as intubation, sedation, hydration, and cooling. Ultimately, the patient fully recovered and was discharged home. This case demonstrates the misconception by the public regarding the safety of synthetic drugs, like N-BOMB, but gives providers good insight into some of clinical effects associated with newer synthetic drugs.

Specialty-Specific Guidance

Internal Medicine/Family Medicine

- Be aware that newer recreational drugs of abuse have varying degrees of stimulant, dopaminergic, and serotonergic properties.
- Consider these drugs, especially N-BOMB and its derivatives in young patients with new onset of status epilepticus.
- Council patients on the dangers of using such designer drugs.
- Look for signs of serotonin toxicity and if present, be cognizant of avoiding other serotonergic agents during hospitalization (e.g., fentanyl, SSRI).
- Standard urine drug screens will not detect the use of newer designer drugs.
- Aggressive supportive care including high dose benzodiazepines, cooling measures, and occasionally intubation with sedation/paralysis is required to control both agitation and hyperthermia.

Pediatrics

- Be aware that newer recreational drugs of abuse have varying degrees of stimulant, dopaminergic, and serotonergic properties.
- Consider these drugs, especially N-BOMB and its derivatives in young patients with new onset of status epilepticus.
- Council pre-teens and adolescents on the dangers of using such designer drugs.
- Look for signs of serotonin toxicity and if present, be cognizant of avoiding other serotonergic agents during hospitalization (e.g., fentanyl, SSRI).
- Standard urine drug screens will not detect the use of newer designer drugs.
- Aggressive supportive care including high dose benzodiazepines, cooling measures, and occasionally intubation with sedation/paralysis is required to control both agitation and hyperthermia.

Emergency Medicine

- Aggressive supportive care including high dose benzodiazepines, cooling measures, and occasionally intubation with sedation/paralysis is required to control both agitation and hyperthermia.
- IV fluids are important as often these patients have dehydration, hyperthermia, and rhabdomyolysis. For patients with hyperthermia, cold fluids are preferred.
- Standard urine drug screens will not detect the use of newer designer drugs.
- Look for signs of serotonin toxicity and if present, be cognizant of avoiding other serotonergic agents during hospitalization (e.g., fentanyl, SSRI).
- Sometimes, a cluster of similar cases will occur surrounding a festival or other event.

Toxicology

- Be aware that newer recreational drugs of abuse have varying degrees of stimulant, dopaminergic, and serotonergic properties.
- Sometimes, a cluster of similar cases will occur surrounding a festival or other event.
- Consider these drugs, especially N-BOMB in young patients with new onset of status epilepticus.
- Aggressive supportive care including high dose benzodiazepines, cooling measures, and occasionally intubation with sedation/paralysis is required to control both agitation and hyperthermia.
- IV fluids are important as often these patients have dehydration, hyperthermia, and rhabdomyolysis. For patients with hyperthermia, cold fluids are preferred.
- Look for signs of serotonin toxicity and if present, be cognizant of avoiding other serotonergic agents during hospitalization (e.g., fentanyl, SSRI).
- Cyproheptadine has been used with varying success in patients with symptoms of serotonin syndrome/toxicity.
- Confirmatory testing can be obtained from urine or blood using liquid chromatography with tandem mass spectrometry (LC/MS/MS), but may not detect all analogs and will not return in a timely manner to affect clinical care.

Neurology

- Be aware that newer recreational drugs of abuse have varying degrees of stimulant, dopaminergic, and serotonergic properties.
- Consider these designer drugs, especially N-BOMB in young patients with new onset of status epilepticus.
- Standard urine drug screens will not detect the use of newer designer drugs but send out testing is available for many of these agents.
- Aggressive supportive care including high dose benzodiazepines, IV fluids, cooling measures, and occasionally intubation with sedation/paralysis is required.
- Cyproheptadine has been used with varying success in patients with symptoms of serotonin syndrome/toxicity.

References

Aksakal E, Bakirci EM, Emet M, Uzkeser M. Complete atroventricular block due to overdose of pregabalin. Am J Emerg Med. 2012;30(9):2101.

Curry SC, Kashani JS, LoVecchio F, Holubek W. Intraventricular conduction delay after bupropion overdose. J Emerg Med. 2005;29(3):299–305.

Davidson J. Seizures and bupropion: a review. J Clin Psychiatry. 1989;50(7):256–61.

Forrester MB. NBOMe designer drug exposures reported to texas poison centers. J Addict Dis. 2014;33(3):196–201.
Gorodetsky RM, Wiegand TJ, Kamali M. Seizures in the setting of large Pregabalin overdose. Clin Toxicol. 2012;50(4):322.
Hill S, Sikand H, Lee J. A case report of seizure induced by bupropion nasal insufflation. J Clin Psychiatry. 2007;9(1):67–9.
Hill SL, Doris T, Gurung S, Katabe S, Lomas A, et al. Severe clinical toxicity associated with analytically confirmed recreational use of 25I-NBOMe: case series. Clin Toxicol (Phila). 2013;51(6):487–92.
Johnson RD, Botch-Jones SR, Flowers T, Lewis CA. An evaluation of 25B-, 25C, 25D-, 25H-, 25I and 25T2-NBOMe via LC-MS-MS: method validation and analyte stability. J Anal Toxicol. 2014;38(9):479–84.
Kim D, Steinhart B. Seizures induced by recreational abuse of bupropion tablets via nasal insufflation. CJEM. 2010;12(2):158.
Laskowski LK, Elbakoush F, Calvo J, Exantus-Bernard G, Fong J, et al. Evolution of the NBOMes: 25C- and 25B- Sold as 25I-NBOMe. J Med Toxicol. 2014;11(2):237–41.
Lawn W, Barratt WM, Horne A, Winstock A. The NBOMe hallucinogenic drug series: patters of use, characteristics of users and self-reported effects in a large international sample. J Psychopharmacol. 2014;28(2):780–8.
Nielsen LM, Holm NB, Leth-Petersen S, Kristensen JL, Olsen L, Linnet K. Characterization of the hepatic cytochrome P450 enzymes involved in the metabolism of 25I-NBOMe and 25I-NBOH. Drug Test Anal. 2017;9(5):671–9.
Papoutsis I, Nikolaou P, Stefanidou M. 25B-NBOMe and its precursor 2C-B: modern trends and hidden dangers. Forensic Toxicol. 2015;33:1–11.
Poklis JL, Clay DJ, Poklis A. High-performance liquid chromatography with tandem mass spectrometry for the determination of nine hallucinogenic 25-NBOMe designer drugs in urine specimens. J Anal Toxicol. 2014a;38(3):113–21.
Poklis JL, Nanco CR, Troendle MM, Wolfe CE, Poklis A. Determination of 4-bromo-2,5-dimethoxy-N-[(2-methoxyphenyl)methyl]-benzeneethanamine (25B-NBOMe) in serum and urine by high performance liquid chromatography with tandem mass spectrometry in a case of severe intoxication. Drug Test Anal. 2014b;6(7–8):764–9.
Poklis JL, Raso SA, Alford KN, Poklis A, Peace MR. Analysis of 25I-NBOMe, 25B-NBOMe, 25C-NBOMe and other dimethoxyphenyl-N-[(2-methoxyphenyl)methyl]ethanamine derivatives on blotter paper. J Anal Toxicol. 2015;39(8):617–23.
Reedy SJ. Pregabalin overdose. Reactions Weekly. 2010;1328(1):37.
Reedy S, Schwartz M. A case series of recreational pregabalin overdose resulting in generalized seizures. Clin Toxicol. 2010;48(6):616–7.
Rose SR, Poklis JL, Poklis A. A case of 25I-NBOMe (25-I) intoxication: a new potent 5-HT2A agonist designer drug. Clin Toxicol(Phila). 2013;51(3):174–7.
Schifano F, D'Offizi S, Piccione M, Corazza O, Deluca P, et al. Is there a recreational misuse potential for pregabalin? Analysis of anecdotal online reports in comparison with related gabapentin and clonazepam data. Psychother Psychosom. 2011;80(2):118–22.
Stellpflug SJ, Kealey SE, Hegarty CB, Janis GC. 2-(4-Iodo-2,5-dimethoxyphenyl)-N-[(2-methoxypheyl)methyl]ethanamine (25I-NBOMe): clinical case with unique confirmatory testing. J Med Toxicol. 2014;10(1):45–50.
Suzuki J, Poklis JL, Polkis A. "My friend said it was good LSD." A suicide attempt following analytically confirmed 25I-NBOMe Ingestion. J Psychoactive Drugs. 2014;46(5):379–82.
Storrow AB. Bupropion overdose and seizure. Am J Emerg Med. 1994;12(2):183–4.
Tang MH, Ching CK, Tsui MS, Chu FK, Mak TW. Two cases of severe intoxication with analytically confirmed use of the novel psychoactive substances 25B-NBOMe and 25C-NBOMe. Clin Toxicol (Phila). 2014;52(5):561–5.
Zuba D, Sekula K. Analytical characterization of three hallucinogenic N-(2-methoxy)benzyl derivatives of the 2C-series of phenylethylamine drugs. Drug Test Anal. 2013a;5:634–45.
Zuba D, Sekula K, Buczek A. 25C-NBOMe-new potent hallucinogenic substance identified on the drug market. Forensic Sci Internl. 2013b;227:7–14.

Case 11
An Acute Medical Condition in a Patient with Opiate Dependence

1. What are the currently available treatment options for long-term management of opiate dependence?
2. What treatment options exist to treat opioid withdrawal while in the hospital?
3. What is the difference between a pure opiate agonist, an antagonist, and a partial agonist/partial antagonist?
4. What treatment options are available for the patient with acute pain who is on buprenorphine or methadone maintenance?

Abstract Buprenorphine is a partial opiate agonist, which is commonly used for the long-term management of opiate dependence. The timing of when to start buprenorphine, as well as how to treat acute pain crises in individuals on buprenorphine can be difficult. This case highlights some of the challenges in treating patients with acute painful conditions, who are chronically on buprenorphine. In addition, a discussion on other outpatient management strategies and opiate withdrawal ensues.

Keywords Buprenorphine • Opiate dependence • Pain management

History of Present Illness

A 43-year-old male presented to the emergency department with a 1-day history of left lower extremity pain, edema, and shortness of breath. He also complained of chest pain. He was recently diagnosed with a deep vein thrombosis in his left leg and had been on warfarin for this, but ran out of his medications approximately 10 days prior to coming to the ED. He had a history of opioid dependence with previous intranasal heroin abuse, and a prior deep vein thrombosis, diagnosed approximately 3 months prior.

L.R. Dye et al. (eds.), *Case Studies in Medical Toxicology*,
DOI 10.1007/978-3-319-56449-4_11

The patient reported that he had been using 2–3 buprenorphine/naloxone tablets daily, which had been purchased illicitly, on the street. He was non-compliant with his Coumadin regimen.

The patient rated his pain as a 7 on a 1–10 scale, pleuritic, and it was centered in his chest and in his left leg.

Past Medical History	Deep vein thrombosis, L leg
Medications	Non-compliant with warfarin. Illicitly purchasing buprenorphine/naloxone 8/2 mg tablets; 2–3 tablets daily
Allergies	No known drug allergies
Family History	"Catastrophic Antiphospholipid antibody syndrome"
Social History	Past intranasal heroin

Physical Examination

Blood pressure	**Heart rate**	**Respiratory rate**	**O_2 saturation**
108/69 mmHg	106–131 bpm	22 breaths/min	97% on 2 L NC

General: uncomfortable, anxious, and flushed
Skin: pink, warm, asymmetric left lower extremity

Diagnostic Testing

Na	**K**	**Cl**	**CO_2**	**BUN**	**Cr**	**Glucose**
135 mmol/L	3.8 mmol/L	104 mmol/L	18 mmol/L	21 mg/dL	1.1 mg/dL	143 mg/dL

PT	**INR**	**PTT**
13.8 s	1.1	29.2

Ancillary Testing

- Urine drug screen: positive for THC. Negative for opiates, benzodiazepines, cocaine, and amphetamines
- Lower extremity duplex ultrasound: Extensive deep venous thrombus involving the common iliac vein to the popliteal vein, which is unchanged from the prior study.

- CT Angiogram of the chest: Multiple bilateral pulmonary emboli (PE), including the right and left main pulmonary artery; the clot burden has increased since the previous angiogram. There is extension of the pulmonary emboli into the segmental branches of the left upper lobe, right middle lobe, and right upper lobe. There is straightening of the intraventricular septum which indicates some right heart strain.

Initial Treatment

The patient received 18,000 units of subcutaneous dalteparin and 8 mg of warfarin while in the Emergency Department. He was also seen by Medical Toxicology and assessed for opioid withdrawal and dependence and given a buprenorphine/naloxone tablet (8 mg/2 mg) sublingually while in the emergency department.

Hospital Course

The patient was admitted and treated with dalteparin and warfarin for his acute on chronic venous thromboembolism and pulmonary emboli. He was given Suboxone™ (buprenorphine/naloxone). The buprenorphine/naloxone was continued using 4/1 mg dose increments every 6 h while he was experiencing pain from his PE and DVT. He also received intravenous toradol and oral acetaminophen for his pain. On the third hospital day, the patient was switched to a twice daily buprenorphine/naloxone regimen using an 8/2 mg dose.

The patient agreed to follow-up in an outpatient chemical dependency (CD) program and also signed a pain management contract for follow-up in the buprenorphine clinic, which stipulated he would take the buprenorphine appropriately, not divert any buprenorphine, not take additional opiates, and attend the chemical dependency program. He was given a bridge prescription of 14 days of an 8/2 mg dose of buprenorphine/naloxone for twice daily dosing.

What Are the Currently Available Treatment Options for Long-Term Management of Opiate Dependence?

Methadone and buprenorphine are available for opioid treatment of opioid use disorder, and naltrexone is available in both tablet and intramuscular depot form (Vivitrol™) as an antagonist therapy. Methadone is available through federally sanctioned Opioid Treatment Programs (OTP). An OTP can also provide buprenorphine but the vast majority of OTPs provide only methadone. While buprenorphine is available in certain OTPs, most of it is prescribed by individual physician providers, who have obtained a special certification to use it to treat opioid dependence, out of their clinics. The certification is called an "X-waiver certification," and it is an additional DEA number for use when prescribing opioids for the treatment of opioid dependence. To obtain an X-waiver, a physician must take an 8 h training course on opioid dependence and buprenorphine and pass a test related to this material. After this, a Notification of Intent is submitted to the Centers for Substance Abuse Treatment (CSAT). The X-waiver certification is sent to the physician following the Notification submission to CSAT. Individual physicians are limited to 30 unique patients at any given time for their first year of treating opioid dependence, after which they can submit a second notification and attestation in order increase this limit to 100 patients. Physicians who have an X-waiver can apply to the Substance Abuse and Mental Health Services Administration (SAMHSA) to increase the patient limits. Naltrexone can be prescribed by any physician without requiring X-waiver or other certification. Vivitrol™ is provided in monthly depot injections. In addition, there is now a buprenorphine implant available, for patients on stable doses of 8 mg per day or less. The implant is designed to remain in the body for 6 months.

In a hospital setting, when a patient has opioid use disorder in addition to a primary medical condition, the X-waiver certification is not required to provide either buprenorphine or methadone for the treatment of opioid dependence (Laes and Wiegand 2016).

What Treatment Options Exist to Treat Opioid Withdrawal While in the Hospital?

Opioid withdrawal can be treated using supportive medications or it can be treated using opioid agonists. Opioid agonists may be more appropriate if the patient is severely dependent and has a medical comorbidity that requires attention (e.g., pneumonia or cellulitis).

Some supportive medications include clonidine, diphenhydramine or hydroxyzine, and nonsteroidal anti-inflammatory medications. Clonidine can be administered at a dose of 0.1–0.2 mg orally every 6–8 h. If the patient develops orthostatic symptoms or bradycardia, the clonidine should be held. Dehydration may increase the risk of untoward symptoms from the clonidine. Clonidine has been shown to shorten the duration and severity of opioid withdrawal symptoms when used for this purpose. Additional medications including diphenhydramine (50 mg tabs) or hydroxyzine (50–100 mg tabs) can be used adjunctively with clonidine for anxiety or for the mitigation of allergy-type symptoms sometimes experienced with withdrawal. Nausea can be treated with ondansetron or another antiemetic and myalgias can be treated with a nonsteroidal anti-inflammatory medication (NSAID) such as naproxen or ibuprofen. Specific regimens depend upon which symptoms the patient is experiencing. Loperamide may be administered to help control diarrhea, and dicyclomine (10 mg every 6 h) can be used to help with abdominal cramping.

Besides supportive care using non-opioid agonists, the ED and hospital provider are able to use opioid agonists in an emergency setting or during the hospital treatment of other medical conditions to treat opioid withdrawal. Both buprenorphine and methadone can be used for this purpose. The use of opioid agonists to treat withdrawal may facilitate better compliance and facilitate treatment of a primary medical condition (D'Onofrio et al. 2015; Laes 2016; Liebschutz et al. 2014; Wiegand 2016; Suzuki et al. 2015). Patient satisfaction is often higher with this method. Methadone for this purpose should be started at 5–20 mg depending on the level of severity of opioid withdrawal. A withdrawal scoring system such as the Clinical Opioid Withdrawal score (COWs) can be used for this purpose. For mild withdrawal 5–10 mg of methadone should be effective; for more moderate withdrawal 10–15 mg and for severe withdrawal, 20 mg used. If the withdrawal symptoms are still present 4 h after the methadone dose an additional 5–10 mg (maximum) can be administered up to a total dose of 30 mg/day. Some clinicians recommend that a small intramuscular methadone dose (10 mg) be administered to treat opioid withdrawal instead of an oral dose.

Buprenorphine is a partial opioid agonist that can also be used to treat withdrawal and then continued to prevent craving in the hospital setting (Liebschutz et al. 2014). Depending on the availability and community resources, it may be easier to link patients to office-based opioid treatment programs that provide buprenorphine than it is to link a patient to a methadone program from the Emergency Department or hospital setting. Buprenorphine must be administered when a patient is in active withdrawal in order to avoid an abstinence syndrome or precipitated withdrawal (Laes and Wiegand 2016).

If the patient was using a long-acting opioid agonist (e.g., oxymorphone), at least 24 h should elapse before starting buprenorphine. Similarly, for doses of methadone exceeding 40 mg, additional time must elapse before starting buprenorphine due to the risk of precipitating withdrawal.

A test dose of 2 mg can be used 12–24 h after the patient's last use of a short-acting opioid agonist such as heroin. If methadone or a sustained release or other long-acting opioid agonist (e.g., oxymorphone) was used, at least 24 h should elapse before the use of buprenorphine (Rosado et al. 2007). For doses >40 mg of methadone, additional time must elapse before starting buprenorphine due to the long-acting nature of methadone and risk for precipitating withdrawal which increases with the higher doses of methadone. If the patient tolerates a 2 mg dose of buprenorphine, it can be continued up to 8 mg sublingually twice daily in the hospital setting. If any sedation develops to buprenorphine, or any other opioid agonist, the doses should be held and the patient re-evaluated. The sedation and risk for overdose is much less when using buprenorphine than when using methadone. Buprenorphine has fewer overall side effects than methadone, including less effect on libido. Also, the office-based opioid treatment setting offers fewer rules and regulations for buprenorphine than methadone maintenance (Laes and Wiegand 2016; Mattock et al. 2014; Donaher and Welsch 2006).

What Is the Difference Between a Pure Opiate Agonist, an Antagonist, and a Partial Agonist/Partial Antagonist?

Methadone is a full agonist, buprenorphine a partial agonist, and naltrexone is an antagonist. Opioid substitution is accomplished using either a partial agonist or full agonist. Naltrexone is used only to block the effects of opioids during relapse; however, it doesn't provide the opioid agonist effect which mitigates craving and withdrawal. Use of naltrexone for long-term treatment of opioid dependence is not effective unless used as a depot injection, which eliminates the need for daily dosing, in order to continue the opioid receptor blockade. Both methadone and buprenorphine prevent craving and withdrawal and create tolerance to the effects of opioid activation, limiting the effects of other opioids when they are added to either drug (Mattock et al. 2014). Compared to full agonists such as morphine, methadone, or oxycodone, which have somewhat linear dose-dependent effects at the mu-receptor, buprenorphine only partially activates the mu-receptor. As the buprenorphine concentration at the receptor increases, activation starts to plateau with the drug behaving more like an antagonist. This creates a "ceiling" effect with regard to activity and subsequent clinical effects, including CNS and respiratory depression. Buprenorphine also has a very high affinity for the mu-receptor along with a very slow dissociation from it. These properties allow for blockade when other opioid agonists are administered (Donaher and Welsch 2006; Sporer 2004).

What Treatment Options Are Available for the Patient with Acute Pain Who Is on Buprenorphine or Methadone Maintenance?

There are several different options to treat acute pain in the patient maintained on opioid agonist therapy. The specific treatment depends on the type and location of pain and the familiarity of the clinician with the specific and nuanced pharmacology of methadone or buprenorphine and the particular type of opioid agonist therapy a patient is receiving.

For all patients, non-opioid analgesic options should be maximized including use of nonsteroidal anti-inflammatory drugs (NSAIDS) such as intravenous ketorolac or use of naproxen or ibuprofen by mouth. Acetaminophen can also be used for acute pain. If the pain is in a digit or extremity, it may be amendable to a nerve block using local anesthetic agents. For severe pain, non-opioid drugs such as ketamine or even general anesthetics such as propofol can provide immediate relief. For less severe pain, muscle relaxants, like benzodiazepines or baclofen, can be added to non-opioid medications. In the methadone-maintained patient, either fentanyl or hydromorphone can be used on top of the patient's maintenance dose of methadone (Laes 2016). The patient's tolerance will limit the effect and duration of the short-acting opioid; however, more frequent dosing and higher dosing amounts can provide effective pain control (Laes and Wiegand 2016; Wiegand 2016). When buprenorphine is being used, it can be switched to more frequent dosing to provide better analgesic coverage. In a patient maintained on 8/2 mg Suboxone™ every 12 h, switching to 4/1 mg sublingual every 6 h will provide better pain control. High doses of potent opioid agonists such as fentanyl, sufentanyl, or hydromorphone can also be used to overcome the "blockade" of buprenorphine. If the pain is transient and self-limited, the doses of buprenorphine can be continued after the short-acting opioid is used. If the pain is severe and is expected to persist, buprenorphine should be discontinued. Patients should be monitored closely for signs of respiratory depression when high doses of full opioid agonists are used in an attempt to overcome the blockade of buprenorphine. Notification of the patient's addiction provider or office-based opioid treatment provider during this time is important to facilitate safe transition, without relapse or other complication, back into their stable maintenance dosing program or regimen (Laes 2016).

Specialty-Specific Guidance

Internal Medicine/Family Medicine

- Commonly used agents for long-term management of opioid dependence include methadone and buprenorphine.
- In order to prescribe buprenorphine, a special "X-waiver certification" is needed from the DEA

Pain Management

- Options for treatment of opioid dependence involving long-acting medications include an extended release naltrexone (Vivitrol™) and a buprenorphine implant.
- The addition of naloxone to buprenorphine (Suboxone™) reduces the desire of crushing the pills with subsequent parenteral administration.

Critical Care Medicine

- Patients with acute pain who are on buprenorphine daily can receive high doses of potent opioid agonists, such as fentanyl, hydromorphone, or sufentanyl. However, careful monitoring for respiratory depression is needed of such an approach is utilized (Laes 2016; Wiegand 2016).

References

D'Onofrio G, O'Connor PG, Pantalon MV, Chawarski MC, Busch SH, Owens PH, Bernstein SL, Fiellin DA. Emergency department-initiated buprenorphine/naloxone treatment for opioid dependence: a randomized clinical trial. JAMA. 2015;313(16):1636–44.

Donaher PA, Welsch C. Managing opioid addiction with buprenorphine. Am Fam Physician. 2006;73(9):1573–8.

Laes JR. The integration of medical toxicology and addiction medicine: a new era in patient care. J Med Toxicol. 2016;12(1):79–81.

Laes JR, Wiegand TJ. Case presentations from the addiction academy. J Med Toxicol. 2016;12(1):82–94.

Liebschutz JM, Crooks D, Herman D, Anderson B, Tsui J, Meshesha LZ, Dossabhoy S, Stein M. Buprenorphine treatment for hospitalized, opioid-dependent patients: a randomized clinical trial. JAMA Intern Med. 2014;174(8):1369–76.

Mattock RP, Breen C, Kimber J, Davoli M. Buprenorphine maintenance versus placebo or methadone maintenance for opioid dependence. Cochrane Database Syst Rev. 2014;2:CD002207.

Rosado J, Walsh SL, Bigelow GE, Strain EC. Sublingual buprenorphine/naloxone precipitated withdrawal in subjects maintained on 100mg of daily methadone. Drug Alcohol Depend. 2007;90(2–3):261–9.

Sporer KA. Buprenorphine: a primer for emergency physicians. Ann Emerg Med. 2004;43(5):580–4.

Suzuki J, DeVido J, Kalra I, Mittal L, Shah S, Zinser J, Weiss RD. Initiating buprenorphine treatment for hospitalized patients with opioid dependence: a case series. Am J Addict. 2015;24(1):10–4.

Wiegand TJ. The new kid on the block-incorporating buprenorphine into a medical toxicology practice. J Med Toxicol. 2016;12(1):64–70.

Case 12
Acute Hepatitis

1. Based on the patient's symptoms and a review of his previous laboratory studies, what hepatic processes are you concerned about?
2. What is the difference between hepatitis and fulminant hepatic failure?
3. What is cholestatic hepatitis?
4. What agents (pharmaceuticals, over-the-counter drugs, supplements, chemicals) are associated with hepatocellular necrosis?
5. What herbal agents or supplements are associated with the development of hepatic necrosis?
6. Which of the patient's herbal supplements was likely the cause of his symptoms?
7. What is the treatment for patients with hepatotoxicity from Chinese skullcap?
8. What is Germander used for and what are some of the signs and symptoms of Germander-related toxicity?
9. Are other species of *Teucrium* associated with similar hepatic effects or are the effects specific to *T. chamaedrys*?
10. What tool can be used for the establishment of causation?
11. What other herbal supplements are associated with hepatotoxicity?
12. What type of injury occurs from pyrrolizidine alkaloids?

Abstract Many exposures can cause liver injury. This case involves a 46-year-old patient with fever, nausea, vomiting, and signs of hepatic injury. In this chapter, we review pharmaceutical and supplement causes of hepatitis and hepatocellular necrosis.

Keywords Cholestatic jaundice • Hepatitis • Herbal products • Supplements • Chinese skullcap

L.R. Dye et al. (eds.), *Case Studies in Medical Toxicology*,
DOI 10.1007/978-3-319-56449-4_12

History of Present Illness

A 46-year-old male presents to the ED after 5 weeks of intermittent episodes of fever, nausea, and vomiting, that resumed the morning of presentation. His maximal temperature during his illness was 40.3 °C (104.5 °F). The patient reports episodes of symptoms that last about 2–3 days and have resulted in multiple ED visits, as well as two previous hospital admissions. He was most recently discharged from the hospital 5 days ago.

During his first admission, he was tested for mononucleosis (negative heterophile antibody test) and blood cultures were drawn with no bacterial growth noted. He was discharged with the diagnosis of a mononucleosis-like illness.

On his second admission, a more extensive workup included testing for human immunodeficiency virus, cytomegalovirus, Epstein–Barr virus, *Borrelia hermseii*, *Bartonella henselae*, malaria, *Leptospira*, and viral hepatitis. None of these tests yielded positive findings. Blood cultures were again repeated, and stool cultures were checked with no abnormalities found. At that time, he was diagnosed with presumptive *Rickettsia* and was started on doxycycline.

Past Medical History	Arthritis Gout
Medications	Move Free® Advanced Montmorency tart cherry capsules Acetaminophen as needed
Allergies	NKDA
Social History	Denies tobacco use Occasional alcohol consumption No other drug use
Family History	Unknown, patient was adopted

Physical Examination

Blood pressure	Heart rate	Respiratory rate	Temperature	O_2 saturation
119/72 mmHg	104 bpm	28 breaths/min	39 °C (102.2 °F)	93% (room air)

General: No acute distress. Well-appearing, well-nourished middle age gentleman
Skin: Warm, dry. No rash
Eyes: Pupils equal, round and reactive to light bilaterally 4 mm to 2 mm
Neck: No meningismus
Cardiovascular: Tachycardic. Normal distal pulses. Normal S1–S2
Pulmonary: Clear to auscultation bilaterally. No tenderness to palpation
Abdomen: Soft, non-tender, non-distended. Present bowel sounds
Extremities: Atraumatic, no edema

Neuro: Awake, alert, and oriented to person, place, time, and situation. Strength 5/5 all extremities. Grossly intact sensation. No tremor

Past Laboratory Studies Available

Liver function tests from second hospitalization:

	Baseline	Day 1 (am)	Day 1 (pm)	Day 2	Day 3	Day 4
AST (U/L)	37	121	75	64	47	36
ALT (U/L)	71	131	96	91	70	58
T Bili (mg/dL)	1	4	2.7	1.9	1.5	1.4
Alk phos (U/L)	85	215	155	151	166	146

Based on the Patient's Symptoms and a Review of His Previous Laboratory Studies, What Hepatic Processes Are You Concerned About?

- Viral hepatitis
- Cholestatic hepatitis
- Hepatocellular necrosis
- Drug-induced hepatitis
- Autoimmune hepatitis

What Is the Difference Between Hepatitis and Fulminant Hepatic Failure?

- Hepatitis
  - Simply put, this is an inflammation of the liver.
  - Hepatitis can result in elevation of aspartate transaminase (AST) and alanine transaminase (ALT), which indicates hepatic injury
- Fulminant hepatic failure, also called acute liver failure
  - Liver injury that progresses to decreased protein synthesis, coagulopathy, and encephalopathy.
  - This term refers to the onset of liver failure with rapid deterioration from the development of jaundice to encephalopathy over days to 2 weeks.
- Some authors report the deterioration that occurs over 8 weeks while others have defined this 8-week time course as late onset hepatic failure.

What Is Cholestatic Hepatitis?

- Cholestatic hepatitis is the impairment of bile synthesis and flow.
  - In this case, cholestatic hepatitis was toxin-induced.
  - This occurs from direct toxin damage to canalicular cells but doesn't always affect hepatocytes (AST and ALT may be normal).
  - Alkaline phosphatase and bilirubin levels are elevated.
- Symptoms and clinical findings often include dark urine, pruritus.
- There is often a period of 2–24 weeks between initial exposure and onset of symptoms.

What Agents (Pharmaceuticals, Over-the-Counter Drugs, Supplements, Chemicals) Are Associated with Hepatocellular Necrosis?

Acetaminophen	Iron	Quinine
Amatoxin	Methotrexate	Sulfonamides
Arsenic–contamination	Methyldopa	Tetrachloroethane
Allopurinol	Nitrofurantoin	Tetracycline
Carbamazepine	Phenytoin	Trinitrotoluene
Carbon tetrachloride	Yellow phosphorus	Troglitazone
Chlordecone	Procainamide	Vinyl Chloride
Hydralazine	Propylthiouracil	

What Herbal Agents or Supplements Are Associated with the Development of Hepatic Necrosis?

- Jin bu wan—tetrahydrapalmatine
- Polar bear livers—vitamin A excess/toxicity
- Chinese skull cap
- Black catechu

Diagnostic Testing

Laboratory Studies from Current Hospitalization

WBC	Hemoglobin	Platelets
8.5 k/mm^3	15.2 g/dL	155 k/mm^3

Na	K	Cl	CO_2	BUN/Cr
139 mmol/L	4.2 mmol/L	102 mmol/L	28 mmol/L	10/1.04 mg/dL

Urinalysis: within normal limits
Liver function tests from current hospitalization:

	Day 1	Day 2 (am)	Day 2 (pm)	Day 3	Day 4
AST (U/L)	137	89	99	87	66
ALT (U/L)	55	91	94	120	102
T Bili (mg/dL)	4	2.4	2.9	4.1	1.9
Alk phos (U/L)	83	84	86	98	124

Ancillary Testing

EKG: Normal sinus rhythm with a rate of 96 beats per min, QRS 86 ms, QTc 459 ms.

Hospital Course

Following his second admission, the patient questioned a correlation of his symptoms with the use of herbal supplements. The supplements were the only medications not continued during his admissions and symptoms improved while hospitalized. Additionally, his symptoms recurred after about 2–3 doses of supplement between his first and second admission. On the day of presentation, he noted recurrence of symptoms after only one dose of the supplement. He was again admitted to the hospital and had resolution of symptoms in 3 days. His supplements were discontinued and his liver function tests improved.

Which of the Patient's Herbal Supplements Was Likely the Cause of His Symptoms?

- Move Free® Advanced contains glucosamine, chondroitin, hyaluronic acid, Chinese skullcap, and black catechu.
- There are several cases reported in the literature describing hepatotoxicity from Move Free® Advanced arthritis supplements. These cases link the development of hepatotoxicity with Chinese skullcap (*Scutellaria baicalensis*). (Dhanasekaran et al. 2013; Linnebur et al. 2010; Yang et al. 2012).
- American skullcap containing products have been contaminated with Germander (*Teucrium chamaedrys*), a known hepatotoxin which is very similar in appearance to American skullcap.

- There are some concerns that Germander may be a contaminant in Move Free® Advanced but there was no confirmation of the presence of Germander or Chinese skullcap in this product.
- Montmorency tart cherry capsules are made from concentrated Montmorency cherries, a sour cherry. There are multiple reported health benefits (natural treatment for gout, antioxidant properties, etc.) but no case reports documenting adverse effects.
- It is most likely this patient's hepatotoxicity was related to the Move Free® Advanced arthritis supplements he was taking and it is possible Chinese skullcap was responsible for this.

What Is the Treatment for Patients with Hepatotoxicity from Chinese Skullcap?

- In the cases reported in the literature, discontinuation of the product resulted in resolution of symptoms and normalization of transaminases.
- The time to recovery varies from patient to patient and can be days, weeks, or months.

What Is Germander Used for and What Are Some of the Signs and Symptoms of Germander-Related Toxicity?

- Plants in the genus *Teucrium* are often referred to as germanders. The one specifically named Germander is *Teucrium chamaedrys*.
- Germander (*Teucrium chamaedrys*) is a plant that was sold as a weight loss aid in France.
- It was withdrawn from the market after causing hepatitis in a large number of patients taking this medication for its slimming properties (Gori 2011).
- Due to physical similarities to American skullcap, Germander has been an accidental contaminant in herbal products reported to contain skullcap.
- Hepatitis is the biggest symptom of Germander-related toxicity. Cirrhosis, chronic hepatitis, and fulminant hepatic failure have also been reported (Larrey et al. 1992).
- Recurrence of hepatitis or worse has been noted with re-exposure to Germander (Gori 2011; Larrey et al. 1992; Larrey 1995; Loeper et al. 1994).
- Other more ambiguous symptoms include nausea, vomiting, anorexia, and abdominal pain.

Are Other Species of Teucrium *Associated with Similar Hepatic Effects or Are the Effects Specific to* T. chamaedrys*?*

- Hepatic dysfunction has been associated with *T. polium*, *T. capitatum*, and *T. viscidium*

- *Teucrium polium*
  - Used as an herbal medication to treat diabetes mellitus and fever, cases of cholestatic hepatitis and hepatocellular injury have been reported with *T. polium* (Mazokopakis et al. 2004; Starakis et al. 2006)
  - There is a case report documenting fulminant hepatic failure requiring transplant (Mattei et al. 1995)
- *Teucrium capitatum* (Dourakis 2002)
  - In this case, the patient had been drinking a tea of *T. capitatum* daily for 4 months to treat hyperglycemia
- *Teucrium viscidum*
  - Used in Chinese herbal medicine to treat low back pain, one patient developed cholestatic hepatitis (Poon 2008).
  - Gas chromatography of the herb used identified the presence of teucvin, a furoano neoclerodane diterpnoid found in *T. viscidum*. Teucvin is structurally similar to teucrin, the neoclerodane diterpenoid thought to be responsible for hepatotoxicity caused by *T. chamaedrys*.

What Tool Can Be Used for the Establishment of Causation?

The Bradford-Hills Criteria was published in 1965 as a list of nine measures that aid in determining whether there is causality to an association. These include:

- Strength of Association
  - A strong association as determined by risk, more likely suggests a causal relationship.
- Consistency
  - Relationship between events is observed repeatedly.
- Specificity
  - Degree to which an exposure leads to an outcome.
- Temporality
  - Exposure must occur prior to the development of the expected outcome.
- Biological gradient
  - The higher the exposure the more the outcome is likely.
- Plausibility
  - The association has a biologically plausible mechanism.

- Coherence
  - The association does not contradict previously established knowledge.
- Experiment
  - Causation is more likely if supported by randomized controlled trials.
- Analogy
  - It is reasonable to consider similar exposures leading to similar effects.

Although these considerations were not meant to be criteria in determining causation, over time, they have been used as such in multiple studies (Höfler 2005).

What Other Herbal Supplements Are Associated with Hepatotoxicity?

- Pennyroyal oil (*Hedeoma pulegioides*; *Mentha pulegium*)
- Chaparral (*Larrea tridentate*)
- Germander (*Teucrium chamaedrys*)
- Kava kava (*Piper methysticum*)
- Pyrrolizidine alkaloids
  - Borage aka: *Borago officinalis*
  - Comfrey aka: *Symphytum officinale*

What Type of Injury Occurs from Pyrrolizidine Alkaloids?

- Veno-occlusive disease occurs from pyrrolizidine alkaloids (Ridker and McDermott 1989).
- Veno-occlusive disease results from intimal thickening of the terminal hepatic venules from toxin-induced injury to the endothelium. This results in edema and nonthrombotic obstruction.
- Fibrosis can develop in the central and sublobular veins.
- Sinusoidal dilation in the centrilobular areas is associated with hepatic necrosis and cellular injury.

Case Conclusion

This patient had cholestatic hepatitis, the development of which was associated with use of Move Free® Advanced arthritis supplements. Move Free® Advanced arthritis supplements have been associated with the development of cholestatic hepatitis due to Chinese skullcap. With discontinuation of the product and supportive care, this patient's symptoms resolved, his transaminases returned to baseline, and he was ultimately discharged home.

Specialty-Specific Guidance

Internal Medicine/Family Medicine

- Consider obtaining liver function testing in the setting of fever with nausea and vomiting of unknown etiology, especially if patient returning to your office with symptoms for a second or third time.
- In patients with signs of hepatic injury of unknown etiology consider pharmaceuticals, herbal supplements, and over-the-counter medications.
  - Obtain a complete history of all medicines in the home, including over-the-counter agents, supplements, and herbals medications/remedies.
  - This should include all products taken in the previous three months as there may be prolonged latency with some agents.
  - If pharmaceuticals are suspected, ensure that liver function testing occurs, as it may provide supporting evidence for toxin-induced reactions.
  - Recommend a period of abstinence of non-prescribed medications and/or herbals/supplements until re-evaluated by primary provider or evaluated by specialist.
- Different pharmaceutical, herbal, and over-the-counter agents cause varying degrees of hepatic injury. Early consultation with your local poison control center or toxicologist and thorough medication/supplement history will help identify products may be causing adverse effects. Treatment options will vary depending upon the potential exposure and severity of illness.

Emergency Medicine

- Consider obtaining liver function testing in the setting of fever with nausea and vomiting of unknown etiology.
- Gather a complete history of all medicines in the home that includes over-the-counter agents, supplements, and herbal medications/remedies over the last three months.
- Recommend a period of abstinence of non-prescribed medications or herbals/supplements until evaluated by primary provider or specialist.
- Supportive care and abstinence from the offending agent is the mainstay of treatment for herbal-induced hepatitis.

- Different pharmaceutical, herbal, and over-the-counter agents cause varying degrees of hepatic injury. Early consultation with your local poison center or toxicologist and thorough medication/supplement history will help identify products may be causing adverse effects. Treatment options will vary depending upon the potential exposure and severity of illness. The diagnosis of herbal product-induced hepatitis is a diagnosis of exclusion.

Toxicology

- Evaluate all the available medications, supplements, and over-the-counters available to the patient.
  - Consider potential contamination of herbal supplements or over-the-counter medications as a cause for the presenting symptoms.
  - Explore the literature to evaluate similar case presentations with similar agents.
- If possible, try and obtain some of the product taken by the patient for testing. This may assist in identifying product contamination or ingredient misidentification.
- The diagnosis of herbal product-induced hepatitis is a diagnosis of exclusion.
- Different pharmaceutical, herbal, and over-the-counter agents cause varying degrees of hepatic injury. Treatment options will vary depending upon the potential exposure and severity of illness.

References

Dhanasekaran R, Owens V, Sanchez W. Chinese skullcap in move free arthritis supplement causes drug induced liver injury and pulmonary infiltrates. Case Rep Hepatol. 2013;2013:1–4.

Dourakis SP, et al. Acute hepatitis associated with herb (Teucrium capitatum L.) administration. Eur J Gastroenterol Hepatol. 2002;14:693–5.

Gori L, Galluzzi P, Mascherini V, et al. Two contemporary cases of hepatitis associated with Teucurium chamaedrys L. decoction use: case reports and review of the literature. Basic Clin Pharmacol Toxicol. 2011;109:521–6.

Höfler M. The Bradford Hill considerations on causality: a counterfactual perspective. Emerg Themes Epidemiol. 2005;2:11.

Larrey D, Vial T, Pauwels A, et al. Hepatitis after Germander (Teucrium chamaedrys) administration: another instance of herbal medicine hepatotoxicity. Ann Intern Med. 1992;117:129–32.

Larrey D. Hepatotoxicity of herbal remedies and mushrooms. Semin Liver Dis. 1995;15:183–8.

Loeper J, Descatoire V, Letteron P, Moulis C, Degott C, Dansette P, et al. Hepatotoxicity of Germander in mice. Gastroenterology. 1994;106:464–72.

Linnebur SA, Rapacchietta OC, Vejar M. Hepatotoxicity associated with Chinese skullcap contained in Move Free Advanced dietary supplement: two case reports and review of the literature. Pharmacotherapy. 2010;30:258e–62e.

Mattei A, Rucay P, Samuel D, Feray C, Reyenes M, Bismuth H. Liver transplantation for severe acute liver failure after herbal medicine (Teucrium polium) administration. J Hepatol. 1995;22:597.

Mazokopakis E, Lazarido S, Tzardi M, Mixaki J, Diamantis I, Ganotakis E. Acute cholestatic hepatitis caused by *Teucrium polium* L. Phytomedicine. 2004;11:83–4.

Poon WT, et al. Hepatitis induced by Teucrium viscidum. Clin Toxicol. 2008;46:819–22.

Ridker P, McDermott W. Comfrey herb tea and hepatic veno-occlusive disease. Lancet. 1989;1(8639):657–8.

Starakis I, Siagris D, Leonidou L, Mazokopakis E, Tsamandas A, Karatza C. Heptatitis caused by the herbal remedy *Teucrium polium* L. Eur J Gastroenterol Hepatol. 2006;18:681–3.

Yang L, Aronsohn A, Hart J, Jensen D. Herbal hepatotoxicity from Chinese skullcap: a case report. World J Hepatol. 2012;4(7):231–3.

Case 13
Thyroid Supplement Ingestion

1. What are the symptoms of thyrotoxicosis?
2. How is thyrotoxicosis different from thyroid storm?
3. How do you differentiate between new onset thyroid disease and exogenous thyroid ingestion/misuse?
4. Are there any similarities between thyroid medication and lithium overdose?
5. Is activated charcoal an option to prevent drug absorption with thyroid hormone ingestions?
6. What is the general time frame from ingestion of levothyroxine (T4) to development of symptoms?
7. Is there any role for early laboratory evaluation of acute levothyroxine (T4) or T3 ingestions?
8. What is the standard treatment for chronic or acute ingestion of thyroid hormone resulting in thyrotoxicosis?
9. Why don't we use other medications typically used to treat naturally occurring thyrotoxicosis to treat overdoses?
10. Why is use of propranolol beneficial?
11. What can you use if a beta-blocker is contraindicated (patient is asthmatic)?
12. What are side effects of propranolol use in children should providers be aware of?
13. How is disposition determined after an ingestion of thyroid medication?
14. How do you follow these patients in the hospital and after discharge to ensure improvement?

Abstract This case involves a 2-year-old female who ingested some of her father's prescribed medication. She presented early to the emergency department where she received activated charcoal. On a follow-up call from the local poison control center 3 days later, she had developed vomiting, agitation, and appeared to have increased work of breathing. We review possible causes for the patient's symptoms including thyroid hormone toxicity, lithium toxicity, and management guidelines for her specific overdose.

Keywords Pediatric • Thyroid supplement ingestion • Thyroxine • Propranolol

L.R. Dye et al. (eds.), *Case Studies in Medical Toxicology*,
DOI 10.1007/978-3-319-56449-4_13

History of Present Illness

- A 2-year-old female was brought to the ED within a couple of hours of ingesting her father's medication. An estimated 30–60 tablets were missing.

Past Medical History	None
Medications	None
Allergies	NKDA
Family History	None
Social History	Lives with parents

Physical Examination

Blood pressure	**Heart rate**	**Respiratory rate**	**Weight**
88/55 mmHg	105 bpm	28 breaths/min	10 kg

General: Alert, playful child
Cardiovascular: Normal heart rate with no murmurs, gallops, or rubs noted
Skin: Warm and dry
Neurologic: Normal behavior for age

Hospital Course

- She was given a dose of 1 g/kg AC and discharged home after a 2-h observation period with no changes in vital signs or behavior.

Post-hospital Follow-up

- On routine poison center follow-up 3 days later, the patient's family reported the patient had developed nausea, vomiting with 6–7 episodes of emesis, decreased oral intake, and agitation.
- She seemed to have increased work of breathing over last 6–8 h.
- The patient was sent back to ED for repeat evaluation.

Second Hospital Visit: (3 days After Initial Presentation)

Physical Examination

Blood pressure	Heart rate	Respiratory rate	Temperature
Not recorded	180 bpm	26 breaths/min	36.7 °C (98 °F)

General: The patient was alert and interactive.
HEENT: No pupillary changes.
Pulmonary: Breath sounds clear on auscultation bilaterally.
Neurologic: There was no tremor and she was sitting up playing with toys, moving all four extremities.

Differential Diagnosis

- Thyroid medication ingestion
- Sustained release lithium ingestion
- Possible ingestion of something else since time of original evaluation
  - Stimulant
  - Caffeine
  - Cocaine
  - Liquid nicotine
- Intestinal obstruction from activated charcoal
- Concurrent viral illness

Diagnostic Testing

Na	K	Cl	CO_2	BUN/Cr
139 mmol/L	4.2 mmol/L	103 mmol/L	26 mmol/L	12/0.3 mg/dL

Glucose	Phosphorous
97 mg/dL	2.9 (4.5–5.5 mg/dL)

Ancillary Testing

TSH	Free T4	T3	Free T3
0.04 (0.27–4.2 mIU/L)	>5.7 (0.8–1.9 ng/dL)	274 (80–200 ng/dL)	11.29 (2.44–4.4 pcg/mL)

EKG demonstrated sinus tachycardia with normal axis and intervals.

Hospital Course

- This patient was admitted and placed on telemetry.
- Due to persistent tachycardia the next morning, she was started on 2 mg of oral propranolol every 8 h.
- Her pulse decreased to 100–110 beats/min, she was eating well, never developed tremor or seizures.
- Propranolol was given for 2 days and she was discharged home without a taper.
- Repeat T3 the next day was 9.7 pcg/mL.
- On follow-up remained without symptoms and with continued decrease of T3.

What Are the Symptoms of Thyrotoxicosis?

- Endogenous and exogenous thyroid hormone excess can cause very similar symptoms.
- Increased metabolism resulting in fever, diaphoresis, and weight loss.
- GI symptoms include diarrhea and weight loss despite an increased appetite (although many of reports deal with Graves Disease, rather than acute thyroid medication overdose, where decreased appetite has been reported) (Ho et al. 2011; Lazar et al. 2000).
- Central nervous system effects include agitation and tremor.
- Cardiac effects include tachycardia, dysrhythmias, and high output heart failure.

How Is Thyrotoxicosis *Different from* Thyroid Storm?

- In thyrotoxicosis, the patient is demonstrating signs of toxicity from excess T3 and T4, i.e., hyperthyroidism.
- In thyroid storm, patients have typically had symptoms of hyperthyroidism that are then worsened by some new stressor, like an acute illness.
- When stressed or the hyperthyroidism progresses, patients may develop altered mental status, seizures, coma, and hypotension.
- Endogenous and exogenous thyroid hormone excess can cause very similar symptoms.

How Do You Differentiate Between New Onset Thyroid Disease and Exogenous Thyroid Ingestion/Misuse?

- Patients with thyrotoxicosis and high levels of T3 and T4 with suppressed TSH and low levels of thyroid-binding globulin are likely to have symptoms related to exogenous thyroid hormone ingestion/misuse (Mariotti et al. 1982).

Are There Any Similarities Between Thyroid Medication and Lithium Overdose?

- GI symptoms may be seen in both (nausea, vomiting, diarrhea)
- Course tremor is a prominent finding of lithium toxicity, while a fine tremor is more typical of thyroid hormone excess.
- Neurologic findings such as altered mental status, coma, and seizures are seen within 1–2 days after an acute lithium overdose or as a late feature of chronic excess.
- Cardiac conduction abnormalities are more typical of lithium than thyroid hormone overdose; tachycardia may be seen in both, but would be more pronounced and associated with other sympathomimetic symptoms in thyroid excess.

Is Activated Charcoal an Option to Prevent Drug Absorption with Thyroid Hormone Ingestions?

- Activated charcoal is an option for thyroid hormone ingestions and can be given within 1 h from time of ingestion for maximal effect.
- Thyroid hormone binds to activated charcoal.
- It is easy to reach a 10:1 ratio of activated charcoal: thyroid hormone ingested due to mcg sized tablets
- There are varying recommendations for the administration of activated charcoal for thyroid hormone ingestions. One example is as follows:
  - Age > 12 months and
  - Thyroid hormone ingestion >3 mg should receive <3 mg ingestions should not need as low likelihood of delayed symptoms.

What Is the General Time Frame from Ingestion of Levothyroxine (T4) to Development of Symptoms?

- Most patients do not demonstrate symptoms for 7–10 days after ingestion.
- Case reports do suggest some patients develop symptoms within 2–3 days after large ingestions (Ho et al. 2011; Lewander et al. 1989; Litovitz and White 1985; Mandel et al. 1989).

- In those who develop symptoms, initially mild gastrointestinal symptoms may increase and be associated with irritability. These patients should be evaluated for tachycardia. Those with abnormal vital signs (including any elevated temperature) should be monitored for symptom progression, and treatment considered.
- Patients that have ingested T3 containing products, and not levothyroxine, may develop symptoms within hours of ingestion (Pfizer 2014).

Is There Any Role for Early Laboratory Evaluation of Acute Levothyroxine (T4) or T3 Ingestions?

- Although relatively rapidly absorbed from the GI tract (within a few hours), quantitative T4 measurements do not correlate with symptoms, because of the feedback mechanisms noted below which limit conversion to the active T3 (Kaiserman et al. 1995).
- If there is uncertainty as to the nature of the product (or if a mixture has been ingested—e.g., desiccated thyroid), serial measurements of T3 over a day or two may provide information regarding treatment duration (as noted below).
- If it is unclear that an ingestion has occurred, a T4 in the normal range several hours after the possible ingestion could be reassuring. However, this is not usual clinical practice.

What Is the Standard Treatment for Chronic or Acute Ingestion of Thyroid Hormone Resulting in Thyrotoxicosis?

- Supportive care.
- IV fluids.
- Benzodiazepines for agitation or anxiety (antipsychotics may worsen condition).
- Active cooling, benzodiazepines, and possibly intubation for hyperthermia.
- Beta-blockers (typically propranolol) for tachycardia.
- Acetaminophen for fever can be considered if diagnosis in doubt, however would not be effective for thyrotoxicosis.

Why Don't We Use Other Medications Typically Used to Treat Naturally Occurring Thyrotoxicosis to Treat Overdoses?

- The symptom course is typically short and resolves with ongoing elimination of active thyroid hormone; negative feedback is normally operative, resulting in cessation of endogenous thyroid hormone release.
- In addition, conversion of T4 to "reverseT3" (rT3) can minimize some of the effects of T3 as rT3 binds to thyroid receptors but does not activate them.

Why Is Use of Propranolol Beneficial?

- Propranolol can be used for symptom control (tachycardia and tremor).
- It also decreases peripheral conversion of T4 to T3.
- Propranolol may provide protection from seizures.

What Can You Use If a Beta-Blocker Is Contraindicated (i.e., the Patient Is Asthmatic)?

- Calcium channel blockers can be used (Milner and Goldman 1989).
- While diltiazem has been the focus of most research in thyroxicosis, it has been used for chronic management of thyrotoxic patients. Caution should be used in the acute setting with intravenous calcium channel blockers due to the possibility of excessive peripheral vasodilation (particularly with the dihydropyridine class) (Milner and Goldman 1989).
- Do NOT combine diltiazem (or any calcium channel blocker) with propranolol (or other beta-blocker).

What Are Side Effects of Propranolol Use in Children Should Providers Be Aware of?

- Providers should be very cautious of children who receive propanolol subsequently developing hypoglycemia. This is a direct effect of the propranolol (loss of beta-receptor-mediated glycogenolysis, lipolysis, and gluconeogenesis) and may be exacerbated by decreased oral intake while in hospital setting (Holland et al. 2010).
- Patients should be on cardiac monitoring to ensure no development of significant bradycardia.

How Is Disposition Determined After an Ingestion of Thyroid Medication?

- Accidental ingestions of T4 containing agents in otherwise healthy patients with reliable access to health care can be sent home with strict return precautions.
- If a patient arrives less than an hour after isolated levothyroxine ingestion, it is reasonable to give them activated charcoal and discharge them home.

- Admit any patients with intentional ingestions, or ingestions of combination T3/T4 products for monitoring.
- This guidance also applies to patients on thyroid medication chronically with an acute accidental or intentional overdose.

How Do You Follow These Patients in the Hospital and After Discharge to Ensure Improvement?

- Continuous telemetry should be used for those with significant tachycardia and while assessing the impact of propranolol therapy.
- There is no need for frequent T4 testing once a decreasing trend is documented.
- There is some suggestion that following free T3 levels is a better way of determining improvement (Mandel 1989; Majlesi et al. 2010).
- If free T3 levels are decreasing, then the rate of conversion from T4 to T3 has decreased and is exceeded by the conversion to reverse T3 (RT3) and or endogenous T3 clearance.
- Thus, symptoms should be subsiding and treatment can be discontinued.
- If the patient is discharged the same day, as beta-blocker therapy is discontinued, a follow-up visit in 1–2 days to document weight stability, assess for any recrudescent symptoms, and to document vital signs is reasonable.

Case Conclusion

In this case, the patient ingested her father's levothyroxine and despite receiving activated charcoal shortly after presentation to the ED, developed symptoms of thyroid toxicity. The patient was admitted for observation once symptomatic and T3 levels followed. She did well and was discharged home without noted complication.

Specialty-Specific Guidance

Internal Medicine/Family Medicine

- In general, patients who accidentally or intentionally overdose on thyroid hormone do well.
- Unless T3 is ingested, there is generally a lag time between ingestion and onset of symptoms. In most cases, this is 5–7 days but has been seen as early as 24 h after ingestion.
- Although relatively rapidly absorbed from the GI tract (within a few hours), quantitative T4 measurements do not correlate with symptoms because of the feedback mechanisms noted below which limit conversion to the active T3.

- If there is uncertainty as to the nature of the product (or if a mixture has been ingested—e.g., desiccated thyroid), serial measurements of T3 over a day or two may provide information regarding treatment duration (as noted below).
- If it is unclear that an ingestion has occurred, a T4 in the normal range several hours after the possible ingestion could be reassuring. However, this is not usual clinical practice.
- Follow-up calls 1–2 days and 5–7 days after ingestion seeking any symptoms of vomiting, change in appetite, irritability, or tremor should be followed by an assessment of vital signs in those with symptoms.
- Measurement of serum T4 is not useful in asymptomatic individuals, unless used to document or rule-out ingestion when there is an unclear history.
- General supportive care is the mainstay of treatment and includes propranolol for clinically significant tachycardia, benzodiazepines for agitation, and aggressive cooling measures for hyperthermia.
- Known thyroid hormone overdose or accidental ingestion is the one time where you should ***NOT*** use routine therapies (PTU, methimazole, iodine) other than propranolol for thyroid storm or thyrotoxicosis.

Pediatrics

- In general, patients who accidentally or intentionally overdose on thyroid hormone do well.
- Unless T3 is ingested, there is generally a lag time between ingestion and onset of symptoms. In most cases, this is 5–7 days but has been seen as early as 24 h after ingestion.
- Although relatively rapidly absorbed from the GI tract (within a few hours), quantitative T4 measurements do not correlate with symptoms because of the feedback mechanisms noted below which limit conversion to the active T3.
- If there is uncertainty as to the nature of the product (or if a mixture has been ingested—e.g., desiccated thyroid), serial measurements of T3 over a day or two may provide information regarding treatment duration (as noted below).
- If it is unclear that an ingestion has occurred, a T4 in the normal range several hours after the possible ingestion could be reassuring. However, this is not usual clinical practice.
- Follow-up calls 1–2 days and 5–7 days after ingestion seeking any symptoms of vomiting, change in appetite, irritability, or tremor should be followed by an assessment of vital signs in those with symptoms.
- Measurement of serum T4 is not useful in asymptomatic individuals, unless used to document or rule-out ingestion when there is an unclear history.
- General supportive care is the mainstay of treatment and includes propranolol for clinically significant tachycardia, benzodiazepines for agitation, and aggressive cooling measures for hyperthermia.

Emergency Medicine

- In general, patients who accidentally or intentionally overdose on thyroid hormone do well.
- Unless T3 is ingested, there is generally a lag time between ingestion and onset of symptoms. In most cases, this is 5–7 days but has been seen as early as 24 h after ingestion.
- Although relatively rapidly absorbed from the GI tract (within a few hours), quantitative T4 measurements do not correlate with symptoms because of the feedback mechanisms noted below which limit conversion to the active T3.
- If there is uncertainty as to the nature of the product (or if a mixture has been ingested—e.g., desiccated thyroid), serial measurements of T3 over a day or two may provide information regarding treatment duration (as noted below).
- If it is unclear that an ingestion has occurred, a T4 in the normal range several hours after the possible ingestion could be reassuring. However, this is not usual clinical practice.
- Good supportive care is the mainstay of therapy for symptomatic patients.
- Avoid antipsychotics and preferentially use benzodiazepines for agitation if thyroid hormone overdose suspected
- Be aggressive with cooling measures for hyperthermia. This includes cool saline, cool packs, benzodiazepines to decrease agitation, and intubation with paralysis, as well as sedation if necessary.
- Propranolol is the drug of choice for clinically significant tachycardia. Starting doses of 1–2 mg IV every 10–15 min until desired effect achieved have been used in cases of endogenous thyroid storm in adults. Titration in children can begin at lower doses (e.g., 0.1 mg/kg), monitoring for effect over 10 min before repeating or escalating the dose. Amounts approaching 0.7 mg/kg IV have been used in burn patients (Das and Krieger 1969).
- Known thyroid hormone overdose or accidental ingestion is the one time where you should ***NOT*** use routine therapies (PTU, methimazole, iodine) other than propranolol for thyroid storm or thyrotoxicosis.

Toxicology

- In general, patients who accidentally or intentionally overdose on thyroid hormone do well.
- Unless T3 is ingested, there is generally a lag time between ingestion and onset of symptoms. In most cases, this is 5–7 days but has been seen as early as 24 h after ingestion.
- Asymptomatic patients with small accidental ingestions of levothyroxine or other T4 only preparations can be managed at home in the correct situation (easy access to care, reliable parents/caregiver). In this group of patients, symptoms are unlikely or likely to be minor; laboratory investigations are not necessary.

- Although relatively rapidly absorbed from the GI tract (within a few hours), quantitative T4 measurements do not correlate with symptoms because of the feedback mechanisms noted below which limit conversion to the active T3.
- If there is uncertainty as to the nature of the product (or if a mixture has been ingested—e.g., desiccated thyroid), serial measurements of T3 over a day or two may provide information regarding treatment duration (as noted below).
- If it is unclear that an ingestion has occurred, a T4 in the normal range several hours after the possible ingestion could be reassuring. However, this is not usual clinical practice.
- Good supportive care is the mainstay of therapy for symptomatic patients.
- Avoid antipsychotics and preferentially use benzodiazepines for agitation if thyroid hormone overdose suspected.
- Be aggressive with cooling measures for hyperthermia. This includes cool saline, cool packs, benzodiazepines to decrease agitation, and intubation with paralysis, as well as sedation if necessary.
- Propranolol is the drug of choice for clinically significant tachycardia. Starting doses of 1–2 mg IV every 10–15 min until desired effect achieved have been cases of endogenous thyroid storm in adults. Titration in children can begin at lower doses (e.g., 0.1 mg/kg), monitoring for effect over 10 min before repeating or escalating the dose. Amounts approaching 0.7 mg/kg IV have been used in burn patients (Das and Krieger 1969).
- Known thyroid hormone overdose or accidental ingestion is the one time where you should ***NOT*** use routine therapies (PTU, methimazole, iodine) other than propranolol for thyroid storm or thyrotoxicosis.

References

Cytomel [package insert]. Pfizer, New York. 2014. http://labeling.pfizer.com/ShowLabeling.aspx?id=703. Accessed 28 Apr 2015.

Das G, Krieger M. Treatment of thyrotoxic storm with intravenous administration of propranolol. Ann Int Med. 1969;70:985–8.

Ho J, Jackson R, Johnson D. Massive levothyroxine ingestion in a pediatric patient: a case report and discussion. CEJM. 2011;13(3):165–8.

Holland KE, Frieden IJ, Frommelt PC, Mancini AJ, Wyatt D, Drolet BA. Hypoglycemia in children taking propranolol for the treatment of infantile hemangioma. Arch Dermatol. 2010;146(7):775–8.

Kaiserman I, Avni M, Sack J. Kinetics of the pituitary-thyroid axis and the peripheral thyroid hormones in 2 children with thyroxine intoxication. Horm Res. 1995;44(5):229–37.

Lazar I, Kalter-Leibovici O, Pertzelan A, Weintrob N, Josefsberg Z, Phillip M. Thyrotoxicosis in prepubertal children compared with pubertal and postpubertal patients. J Clin Endocrinol Metab. 2000;85:3678–82.

Lewander WJ, Lacouture PG, Silva JE, Lovejoy FH. Acute thyroxine ingestion in pediatric patients. Pediatrics. 1989;84(2):262–5.

Litovitz TL, White JD. Levothyroxine ingestions in children: an analysis of 78 cases. Am J Emerg Med. 1985;3(4):297–300.

Majlesi N, Greller HA, McGuigan MA, Caraccio T, Su MK, Chan GM. Thyroid storm after pediatric levothyroxine ingestion. Pediatrics. 2010;126(2):e470–3. http://pediatrics.aappublications.org/cgi/pmidlookup?view=long&pmid=20643722.

Mandel SH, Magnusson AR, Burton BT, Swanson JR, LaFranchi SH. Massive levothyroxine ingestion. Conservative management. Clin Pediatr. 1989;28(8):374–6.

Mariotti S, Marino E, Cupin C, et al. Low serum thyroglobulin as a clue to the diagnosis of thyrotoxicosis factitia. N Engl J Med. 1982;307:410–2.

Milner MR, Goldman ME. Diltiazem for the treatment of thyrotoxicosis. Arch Intern Med. 1989;149(5):1217.

Case 14
Blue or Rigid: Pick your Toxin

1. What is the mechanism of methemoglobinemia?
2. What is the FDA warning regarding serotonin syndrome and methylene blue?
3. What is the data for serotonin syndrome following methylene blue administration?
4. Besides treatment for methemoglobinemia, what are potential indications for methylene blue?
5. Are there any other potential side effects or adverse events that can be caused by methylene blue?

Abstract Methemoglobinemia is a congenital or acquired hemoglobinopathy caused by abnormal oxidation of hemoglobin. Typically, methemoglobinemia is treated with methylene blue. However, methylene blue is potentially serotonergic, and an FDA warning exists about the possibility of inducing serotonin syndrome. This chapter discusses methemoglobinemia, treatment options for this condition, and adverse reactions associated with methylene blue administration.

Keywords Methemoglobinemia • Serotonin syndrome • Methylene blue

A patient presented to the emergency department in respiratory distress and was diagnosed with pneumonia. The patient was started on antimicrobials and was admitted to the ICU. After admission, the patient again developed respiratory distress, with a saturation of 88%. Ultimately, methemoglobinemia was diagnosed. Concern was raised by the pharmacist regarding the concurrent administration of methylene blue to an individual who is on a selective serotonin reuptake inhibitor. This review discusses these entities.

L.R. Dye et al. (eds.), *Case Studies in Medical Toxicology*,
DOI 10.1007/978-3-319-56449-4_14

Intensive Care Unit

History of Present Illness

A 65-year-old female with a history of depression and breast cancer presented to the emergency department in respiratory distress. Initial thoracic imaging revealed bilateral infiltrates. She was started on broad spectrum antibiotics and admitted to the intensive care unit. Infectious disease consult was obtained, and the patient's antimicrobial coverage was changed to primaquine for possible *pneumocystis jirovecii* pneumonia. The patient clinically improved until hospital day 1, when she developed increasing respiratory distress.

Past Medical History	Breast cancer Depression
Medications	Sertraline Chemotherapy regimen includes doxyrubicin and cyclophosphamide
Allergies	No known drug allergies
Family History	Reviewed and noncontributory

Physical Examination

Blood pressure	Heart rate	Respiratory rate	O_2 saturation
110/80 mmHg	110 bpm	22 breaths/min	88% (on 15 L/min)

General: Sitting upright in bed in moderate acute distress
Pulmonary: Tachypnic. Speaking 3–4 word sentences. Scattered crackles
Cardiovascular: Tachycardic with a regular rhythm. No murmurs appreciated
Neurologic: Awake. Oriented appropriately
Extremity: No edema
Skin: Perioral cyanosis noted

Diagnostic Testing

WBC	Hemoglobin	Platelets
14 k/mm^3	11 g/dL	352 k/mm^3

Na	K	Cl	CO2	BUN	Cr	Glucose
140 mmol/L	4.1 mmol/L	109 mmol/L	20 mmol/L	13 mg/dL	1.3 mg/dL	102 mg/dL

AST	ALT
25 IU/L	23 IU/L

Co-oximetry revealed a methemoglobin concentration of 20%.

Case Continuation

Despite discontinuing primaquine, a repeat methemoglobin concentration was 20%, and she continues to appear cyanotic with pulse oximetry as low as 86%. Methylene blue was ordered, but the pharmacist was concerned over the possibility of administering methylene blue to a patient on a selective serotonin reuptake inhibitor.

What Is the Mechanism of Methemoglobinemia?

Methemoglobinemia can exist in either congenital or acquired variants. In both situations, a common pathway is noted; oxidation of deoxyhemoglobin with resultant conversion of the ferrous (Fe^{2+}) ion to the ferric (Fe^{3+}) valence (Curry 1982; Levine et al. 2013). In normal conditions, the ferric form is converted back to the oxygen-carrying ferrous form via the enzyme cytochrome b5 reductase (NADH methemoglobin reductase) (Curry 1982; Levine et al. 2013). A second enzyme, nicotinamide adenine dinucleotide phosphate (NADPH) methemoglobin reductase can also reduce methemoglobin (Canning and Levine 2011). However, under routine conditions, NADPH methemoglobin reductase is relatively silent, but assumes a much larger role in the reduction in the setting of methylene blue, which utilizes NADPH formed via the hexose monophosphate shunt to reduce methylene blue to leukomethylene blue, thereby donating an electron to reduce methemoglobin (Canning and Levine 2011).

What Is the FDA Warning Regarding Serotonin Syndrome and Methylene Blue?

In 2011, the United States Food and Drug Administration released a warning that methylene blue could potentially cause serotonin syndrome in patients taking serotonergic psychiatric medications. This warning was issued after a number of cases were submitted to the FDA's Adverse Event Reporting System. The majority of these cases occurred in patients maintained on serotonergic psychiatric medications and then received methylene blue at doses between 3 and 5 mg/kg during parathyroid surgery (Ng et al. 2008; Rowley et al. 2009; Sweet and Standiford 2007).

What Is the Data for Serotonin Syndrome Following Methylene Blue Administration?

The data for serotonin syndrome following methylene blue administration is largely based on case reports. Though it is known that methylene blue is a strong monoamine oxidase inhibitor (Ramsay et al. 2007), there are no large studies that elucidate the risk of developing serotonin syndrome when concomitantly given to patients taking serotonergic psychiatric medications. There is some data that suggests even small doses at 1 mg/kg of methylene blue can potentially precipitate serotonin syndrome in patients concurrently on serotoninergic medications (Gillaman 2011). Given the relatively rare occurrence of this adverse drug effect as well as the difficulty in confirming diagnosis, it is difficult to truly understand risk factors for developing serotonin syndrome. There are no prospective studies that quantify these risks in humans although there are two retrospective reviews that highlight encephalopathic states or serotonin syndrome following methylene blue administration in patients taking serotonergic medications (Sweet and Standiford 2007; Ng and Cameron 2010). Serotonergic agents known to induce serotonin syndrome when concomitantly administered with methylene blue include selective serotonin reuptake inhibitors, selective norepinephrine reuptake inhibitors, and tricyclic antidepressants (Rowley et al. 2009; Sweet and Standiford 2007; Ramsay et al. 2007; Gillaman 2011; Ng and Cameron 2010; Grubb et al. 2012; Larson et al. 2015; Top et al. 2014; Smith et al. 2015).

Besides Treatment for Methemoglobinemia, What Are Potential Indications for Methylene Blue?

While methylene blue is not currently an FDA-approved drug, there are many potential uses. Aside from methemoglobinemia, it is also used to treat vasoplegic syndrome following cardiopulmonary bypass surgery and encephalopathy from ifosfamide. It has also been used to treat hypotensive patients with sepsis and dihydropyridine calcium channel blocker overdose (Dumbarton et al. 2011; Jang et al. 2015; Juffermans et al. 2010; Kirov et al. 2001; Paya et al. 1993). Methylene blue is thought to improve hypotension due to its ability to inhibit nitric oxide synthase, guanylyl cyclase, and free radical formation. Due to these mechanisms, methylene blue has also successfully been used to treat priapism and hepatopulmonary syndrome.

Due to its vibrant blue color, methylene blue is often used in surgical procedures as guides for debridement of tissues, intra-articular injections for evaluation of potential penetrating joint injuries, ureteral evaluation during urological procedures, gland identification during parathyroid surgery, and detecting gastric balloon rupture.

Are There any Other Potential Side Effects or Adverse Events That Can Be Caused by Methylene Blue?

While methylene blue is the treatment of choice for symptomatic methemoglobinemia, it also has the potential to induce methemoglobinemia, particularly when very large doses are administered or if there is an abnormality in the NADPH methemoglobin reductase pathway. Some studies suggest that dosing should not exceed 7 mg/kg to avoid the risk of inducing methemoglobinemia (Howland 2015).

A potential concerning side effect following methylene blue administration is hemolytic anemia. Methylene blue is an oxidizing agent and can cause a Heinz body hemolytic anemia. Patients with glucose 6 phosphate dehydrogenase deficiency are at higher risk of developing hemolysis (Kellermeyer et al. 1962).

Due to its vibrant color, methylene blue can cause skin discoloration, mimicking cyanosis and making it difficult for medical providers to determine if cyanosis is improving. The discoloration can also lead to falsely low pulse oximetry readings.

Newborns are particularly sensitive to methylene blue due to their decreased NADH reductase activity. As a result, very small doses of methylene blue should be used when indicated. There are case reports of intra-amniotic exposure of fetuses to methylene blue which have resulted in skin discoloration, methemoglobinemia, and hemolysis (Albert et al. 2003; Crooks 1982; McEnerney and McEnerney 1983).

Specialty-Specific Guidance

Emergency Medicine

- Methemoglobinemia should be suspected when pulse oximetry provides a reading in the upper 80s (e.g., 85–88%) which does not improve significantly with the administration of oxygen.
- The diagnosis of methemoglobinemia should be performed with co-oximetry.

Hematology

- Cytochrome b5 reductase is the primary enzyme responsible for the reduction of the iron valence in hemoglobin.
- Methylene blue accepts an electron from the hexose monophosphate shunt and can reduce methemoglobin via the enzyme leukomethylene blue.

Critical Care Medicine

- Methylene blue may also be utilized in the treatment of various other conditions, including refractory vasoplegic shock, identification of the parotid glands during neck surgeries, identifying joint penetration, and treatment of ifosfamide encephalopathy.
- Patients with life-threatening methemoglobinemia should be treated with methylene blue, even if on serotonergic agents.

References

Albert M, Lessin MS, Gilchrist BF. Methylene blue: dangerous dye for neonates. J Pediatr Surg. 2003;38(8):1244–5.

Canning J, Levine M. Case files of the medical toxicology fellowship at Banner Good Samaritan Medical Center in Phoenix, AZ: methemoglobinemia following dapsone exposure. J Med Toxicol. 2011;7:139–46.

Crooks J. Haemolytic jaundice in a neonate after intra-amniotic injection of methylene blue. Arch Dis Child. 1982;57(11):872–3.

Curry S. Methemoglobinemia. Ann Emerg Med. 1982;11:214–21.

Dumbarton TC, Minor S, Yeung CK, Green R. Prolonged methylene blue infusion in refractory septic shock: a case report. Can J Anesth. 2011;58(4):401–5.

Gillaman PK. CNS toxicity involving methylene blue: the exemplar for understanding and predicting drug interactions that precipitate serotonin toxicity. J Psychopharmacol. 2011;25(3):429–36. https://doi.org/10.1177/0269881109359098. Epub 2010 Feb 8.

Grubb KJ, Kennedy JL, Begin JD, Groves DS, Kern JA. The role of methylene blue in serotonin syndrome following cardiac transplantation: a case report and review of the literature. J Thorac Cardiovasc Surg. 2012;144(5):e113–6. https://doi.org/10.1016/j.jtcvs.2012.07.030. Epub 2012 Sep 13.

Howland MA. Methylene blue. In: Hoffman RS, Howland MA, Lewin N, Nelson LS, Goldfrank LR, editors. Goldfrank's toxicologic emergencies. 10th ed. New York: McGraw-Hill; 2015.

Jang DH, Donovan S, Nelson LS, Bana TC, Hoffman RS, Chu J. Efficacy of methylene blue in an experimental model of calcium channel blocker-induced shock. Ann Emerg Med. 2015;65(4):410–5. https://doi.org/10.1016/j.annemergmed.2014.09.015. Epub 2014 Oct 23.

Juffermans NP, Vervloet MG, Daemen-Gubbels CRG, Binnekade JM, de Jong M, Groeneveld ABJ. A dose-finding study of methylene blue to inhibit nitric oxide actions in the hemodynamics of human septic shock. Nitric Oxide. 2010;22(4):275–80. Elsevier Inc.

Kellermeyer RW, Tarlov AR, Brewer GJ, Carson PE, Alving AS. Hemolytic effect of therapeutic drugs. Clinical considerations of the primaquine-type hemolysis. JAMA. 1962;180:388–94.

Kirov MY, Evgenov OV, Evgenov NV, Egorina EM, Sovershaev MA, Sveinbjørnsson B, et al. Infusion of methylene blue in human septic shock: a pilot, randomized, controlled study. Crit Care Med. 2001;29(10):1860–7.
Larson KJ, Wittwer ED, Nicholson WT, Price DL, Sprung J. Myoclonus in patient on fluoxetine after receiving fentanyl and low-dose methylene blue during sentinel lymph node biopsy. J Clin Anesth. 2015;27(3):247–51. https://doi.org/10.1016/j.jclinane.2014.11.002. Epub 2014 Dec 11.
Levine M, O'Connor AD, Tasset M. Methemoglobinemia after a mediastinal stab wound. J Emerg Med. 2013;45:e153–6.
McEnerney JK, McEnerney LN. Unfavorable neonatal outcome after intraamniotic injection of methylene blue. Obstet Gynceol. 1983;61(3 Suppl):35S–7S.
Ng BK, Cameron AJ. The role of methylene blue in serotonin syndrome: a systematic review. Psychosomatics. 2010;51(3):194–200. https://doi.org/10.1176/appi.psy.51.3.194.
Ng BK, Cameron AJ, Liang R, Rahman H. Serotonin syndrome following methylene blue infusion during parathyroidectomy: a case report and literature review. Can J Anaesth. 2008;55(1):36–41. https://doi.org/10.1007/BF03017595.
Paya D, Gray GA, Stoclet JC. Effects of methylene blue on blood pressure and reactivity to norepinephrine in endotoxemic rats. J Cardiovasc Pharmacol. 1993;21(6):926.
Ramsay RR, Dunford C, Gillman PK. Methylene blue and serotonin toxicity: inhibition of monoamine oxidase A (MAO A) confirms a theoretical prediction. Br J Pharmacol. 2007;152(6):946–51. Epub 2007 Aug 27.
Rowley M, Riutort K, Shapiro D, Casler J, Festic E, Freeman WD. Methylene blue-associated serotonin syndrome: a 'green' encephalopathy after parathyroidectomy. Neurocrit Care. 2009;11(1):88–93. https://doi.org/10.1007/s12028-009-9206-z. Epub 2009 Mar 5.
Smith CJ, Wang D, Sgambelluri A, Kramer RS, Gagnon DJ. Serotonin syndrome following methylene blue administration during cardiothoracic surgery. J Pharm Pract. 2015;28(2):207–11. https://doi.org/10.1177/0897190014568389. Epub 2015 Jan 22.
Sweet G, Standiford SB. Methylene-blue-associated encephalopathy. J Am Coll Surg. 2007;204(3):454–8.
Top WM, Gillman PK, de Langen CJ, Kooy A. Fatal methylene blue associated serotonin toxicity. Neth J Med. 2014;72(3):179–81.

Case 15
Overdose in a Patient with Parkinson Disease

1. What medications are used to treat Parkinson disease (PD)? What are some associated complications?
2. What is rivastigmine and what is its role in PD?
3. What is the toxidrome associated with carbamate overdose?
4. How should this patient be managed?

Abstract Medical carbamates such as rivastigmine are used to treat dementia associated with Alzheimer and Parkinson disease (PD). Rivastigmine is formulated as a transdermal patch to be removed and re-administered daily. This is a case of a 76-year-old man with a history of PD who presented with signs and symptoms of cholinergic excess after he applied, at once, the entire 40-day supply of rivastigmine patches in error. This case highlights the clinical manifestations associated with medical carbamate overdose and the significant risks associated with prescribing transdermal patches to an elderly patient with dementia.

Keywords Cholinergic toxicity • Carbamates • Parkinson disease • Rivastigmine • Pralidoxime

History of Present Illness

A 76-year-old man with Parkinson disease (PD) and hypertension presented to the ED with acute onset of severe tremulousness, blurred vision, salivation, lacrimation, diffuse muscle aches, and extremity weakness.

L.R. Dye et al. (eds.), *Case Studies in Medical Toxicology*,
DOI 10.1007/978-3-319-56449-4_15

A review of the patient's medication history revealed that he was recently prescribed rivastigmine (13.3 mg/24 h transdermal patch). At bedtime, the evening prior to presentation, the patient applied 40 rivastigmine patches, the entire contents of his new prescription, to his body. Approximately 5 h later, he awoke with the previously described findings, at which point his wife removed the patches and brought him to the ED.

Past Medical History	Parkinson disease (PD)
	Dementia
	Hypertension
	GERD
Medications	Rivastigmine
	Carbidopa/levodopa
	Losartan
	Aspirin
	Naproxen
	Pantoprazole
Allergies	NKDA
Social History	Denies tobacco, ethanol, or other drugs of abuse

Physical Examination

Blood pressure	Heart rate	Respiratory rate	Temperature	O_2 saturation
175/74 mmHg	62 bpm	16 breaths/min	37 °C (98.6 °F)	100% (room air)

General: Patient lying in bed, uncomfortable
Neurologic: Alert and oriented to person and place (baseline?); pupils 3 mm, equal, round, reactive to light; coarse resting tremor, motor strength 2/5 in upper and lower extremities
HEENT: Excessive lacrimation and salivation
Cardiovascular: Regular rate and rhythm, no murmurs
Pulmonary: Clear to auscultation, symmetric breath sounds
Abdominal: Soft, non-tender, normal bowel sounds
Skin: Warm and well perfused; w/o excessive dryness or diaphoresis

ED Management

The patient's skin was cleansed thoroughly with soap and water. Supportive and conservative management with IV fluid hydration and close monitoring was provided. The patient was admitted to the medicine floor.

Key Points of Case

How Does the Pathophysiology of PD Explain How Treatments Are Targeted?

Parkinson disease is a neurodegenerative disorder marked by the destruction of dopaminergic neurons of the substantia nigra. Through complex dopamine (DA) pathways modulated by cholinergic input, the substantia nigra regulates neuronal transmission to and from the basal ganglia. Damage to this important brain structure results in four cardinal parkinsonian motor effects: bradykinesia, resting tremor, muscle rigidity, and impairment of postural balance. Together these abnormalities cause gait disturbance and lead to frequent falls. To a lesser extent, PD involves other brain structures, including the brainstem, hippocampus, and neocortex, which likely contribute to the non-motor features of the disease (e.g., sleep disorders, depression, memory impairment). The goal of medical therapy is thus to slow the progression of both motor and cognitive effects (Standaert and Roberson 2011).

What Medications Are Used to Treat PD? What Are some Associated Complications?

There are two broad categories of medications used to treat the motor effects of PD. The majority of these drugs enhance dopaminergic function and improve motor function, while a smaller number block the effects of acetylcholine (ACh) to enhance cognitive function.

Dopamine Precursors and Agonists

Dopamine precursors such as levodopa (l-dopa) can be combined with the l-amino acid decarboxylase inhibitor carbidopa to prevent peripheral metabolism by this enzyme and thereby increase brain concentrations of DA following metabolism by DA decarboxylase in the central nervous system (CNS) (Standaert and Roberson 2011). Dopamine agonists, including bromocriptine, ropinirole, and pramipexole, do not depend on endogenous conversion to DA and have substantially longer durations of action, limiting the dose-related fluctuations in motor function common in some PD patients taking l-dopa (Standaert and Roberson 2011). For these reasons, DA agonists have often replaced l-dopa as initial treatment, especially in younger patients. Catechol-O-methyltransferase inhibitors (tolcapone, entacapone) prevent peripheral breakdown of DA, allowing a higher fraction to reach the CNS. With respect to side effects, all of the dopaminergic medications can cause nausea, hallucinations, confusion, and orthostatic hypotension.

Anticholinergic Drugs

Although the precise mechanism by which anticholinergic drugs improve PD is not fully understood, agents such as trihexyphenidyl, benztropine mesylate, and diphenhydramine hydrochloride were prescribed even before the discovery of l-dopa and continue to be used today (Standaert and Roberson 2011). Adverse effects are a function of the anti-muscarinic (anticholinergic) properties of the drugs and may include mydriasis and blurred vision, dry flushed skin, tachycardia, hyperthermia, constipation, urinary retention, and altered mental status.

Amantadine

In addition to the anticholinergics, amantadine is also used to treat PD. This antiviral agent alters DA release in the brain, produces anticholinergic effects, and blocks N-methyl-d-aspartate glutamate receptors (Standaert and Roberson 2011). Common adverse drug effects include anticholinergic signs as well as nausea, vomiting, dizziness, lethargy, and sleep disturbance, all of which are usually mild and reversible.

What Is Rivastigmine and What Is Its Role in PD?

Rivastigmine is a carbamate-type cholinesterase inhibitor (CEI) indicated for the treatment of mild-to-moderate dementia associated with PD and Alzheimer disease (Rösler et al. 1999). Tacrine, a medicinal noncarbamate CEI, is also prescribed for this use. Both drugs increase ACh concentrations in relevant brain regions and foster the formation of new memory.

Cholinesterase inhibitors are mechanistically analogous to the insecticidal carbamates (e.g., aldicarb) and the organophosphates (OPs) (e.g., malathion). They inhibit the metabolism of ACh by acetylcholinesterase (AChE) in the various cholinergic synapses, increasing the intrasynaptic concentration of ACh. Additional AChEs include physostigmine, a carbamate commonly used in the ED to treat anticholinergic toxicity. Physostigmine raises the local synaptic concentration of ACh to compete for the muscarinic ACh receptor with drugs such as diphenhydramine or atropine. Other CEIs (e.g., neostigmine, pyridostigmine, edrophonium) are used to raise intrasynaptic ACh concentrations and overcome antibody blockade of nicotinic ACh receptors at the neuromuscular junction in patients with myasthenia gravis.

Rivastigmine is formulated as a novel transdermal matrix patch, available in three different daily doses, and prescribed as a monthly supply of patches. It is the first patch-formulated medication available for Alzheimer disease (Kurz et al. 2009).

Due to the potential for error in administering an uncommon formulation of a drug indicated for patients with cognitive impairment, exceptional care must be taken to adequately educate patients and caregivers of the appropriate technique for administration and removal, along with the signs and symptoms of overdose. According to the package insert, one patch should be applied and replaced once every 24 h to clean, dry, hairless, intact health skin (Exelon™) patch (package insert 2013). Recommended sites for application include the upper or lower back, upper arm or chest; sites should not be reused within 14 days.

What Is the Toxidrome Associated with Carbamate Overdose?

The cholinergic toxicologic syndrome is expected following excessive use of a carbamate, whether insecticidal or medicinal. Effects can be categorized by autonomic division, cholinergic receptor, and associated organ systems involved, and vary somewhat among patients. In the parasympathetic division of the autonomic nervous system, agonism of pre-ganglionic nicotinic receptors and post-ganglionic muscarinic receptors produce effects such as salivation, lacrimation, urination, defecation, gastrointestinal upset, and emesis. Miosis, bradycardia, bronchoconstriction, and bronchorrhea can result. In the sympathetic division, agonism of pre-ganglionic nicotinic receptors causes catecholamine release that can produce hypertension, tachycardia, and mydriasis. Stimulation of nicotinic receptors at the neuromuscular junction produces fasciculations and muscle weakness that can progress to paralysis. Stimulation of receptors in the CNS may result in altered mental status, seizure, and/or coma.

Carbamate toxicity, as manifested by the cholinergic toxidrome, largely resembles.

OP toxicity but with an important difference: Both OPs and carbamates function by binding to and inhibiting AChE; however, the carbamate-AChE bond undergoes spontaneous hydrolysis, thereby reactivating the enzyme. Consequently, the clinical effects of carbamate toxicity, though potentially severe, are self-limited and typically last 24 h or less (Eddleston and Clark 2011).

How Should This Patient Be Managed?

The general approach to a patient with medical carbamate toxicity is similar to that of a patient with OP poisoning. Dermal exposure, as in this patient, should prompt skin decontamination to minimize ongoing exposure. Patch removal is necessary but is not sufficient to prevent ongoing absorption since a depot of medication typically forms in the dermal tissue. In the presence of significant or life-threatening muscarinic effects (e.g., bronchorrhea, bronchospasm, seizure), an anti-muscarinic agent such as atropine is indicated. Various dosing schemes of atropine exist; an initial dose of 1–3 mg intravenously (IV), with escalating doses every 5 min until reversal of bronchorrhea and bronchospasm occur (Eddleston and Clark 2011). This is followed by initiation of an atropine infusion at a rate of 10% to 20% of the total loading dose per hour (to a maximum of 2 mg/h).

Pralidoxime (2-PAM) and other oximes accelerate the reactivation of carbamate-inhibited AChE and have effects at both the nicotinic and muscarinic synapses. Reactivation results in the enhanced metabolism of intrasynaptic ACh and decreased clinical cholinergic effects. Since atropine is only effective at muscarinic receptors, oximes were administered in this case (see below) to reverse neuromuscular weakness.

Although early administration of 2-PAM is indicated in the setting of significant OP poisoning (due to irreversible inhibition of AChE), its use for medical carbamate toxicity is controversial. Early animal studies of carbamate toxicity suggested that treatment with oximes worsened outcomes; however, this has not been demonstrated in more recent studies (Natoff and Reiff 1973; Mercurio-Zappala et al. 2007). Therefore, although 2-PAM may be beneficial in treating cases of clinically significant carbamate poisoning (which can be prolonged and severe), these benefits should be weighed against the potential risks.

Case Conclusion

Twelve hours after the onset of symptoms, the patient continued to exhibit profound extremity weakness with no improvement. The Poison Control Center was consulted and advised administration of pralidoxime 1 g IV over 30 min. Shortly thereafter, patient's motor strength improved from 2/5 to 3/5 in both upper and lower extremities. No complications were noted, and the patient's weakness and tremulousness continued to resolve. He was transferred to a skilled nursing facility on hospital day six.

Specialty-Specific Guidance

Internal Medicine/Family Medicine

- When prescribing patch medications to patients, ensure an adequate understanding, from the patient or caregiver, of appropriate patch administration and removal.
- When prescribing a medical carbamate, advise your patient on the cholinergic effects which may arise with drug misuse.
- In patients admitted to the hospital with a drug-related complaint, be sure to consult a medical toxicologist.

Emergency Medicine

- Remember the cholinergic toxidrome:
  - Muscarinic findings (mnemonic: SLUDGE and the 3 Killer Bs):

    Salivation
    Lacrimation
    Urination
    Defecation
    GI upset
    Emesis
    Bradycardia
    Bronchorrhea
    Bronchoconstriction
    Miosis

  - Nicotinic findings

    Muscle weakness
    Fasciculations
    Mydriasis
    Proptosis

- ED management of the patient with cholinergic toxicity from carbamates includes:
  - early recognition
  - skin and/or clothing decontamination
  - careful handling to avoid secondary contamination of healthcare personnel
  - aggressive supportive care
  - atropine:

    initial dose: 1–3 mg intravenously (IV)
    double dose: q 5 min until reversal of bronchorrhea and bronchospasm
    maintenance dose: 10% to 20% of the total loading dose per hour

      maximum of 2 mg/h

    indications for administration of atropine include:

      Bradycardia
      Bronchorrhea
      Bronchoconstriction

Toxicology

- In patients with severe cholinergic toxicity due to a medical carbamate who exhibit significant nicotinic effects, consider:
  - pralidoxime:

    initial dose: 1–2 g in 100 mL of 0.9% NaCl IV over 15–30 min
    repeat dose: may repeat initial dose at 3 h if symptoms severe or recur

References

Eddleston M, Clark RF. Insecticides: organic phosphorus compounds and carbamates. In: Nelson LS, Lewis NA, Howland MA, Hoffman RS, Goldfrank LR, Flomenbaum NE, editors. Goldfrank's toxicologic emergencies. 9th ed. New York: McGraw-Hill; 2011. p. 1450–66.

Exelon™ Patch [package insert]. East Hanover. NJ: Novartis Pharmaceuticals Corporation; 2013.

Kurz A, Farlow M, Lefevre G. Pharmacokinetics of a novel transdermal rivastigmine patch for the treatment of Alzheimer's disease: a review. Int J Clin Pract. 2009;63(5):799–805.

Mercurio-Zappala M, Hack JB, Salvador A, Hoffman RS. Pralidoxime in carbaryl poisoning: an animal model. Hum Exp Toxicol. 2007;26(2):125–9.

Natoff IL, Reiff B. Effect of oximes on the acute toxicity of anticholinesterase carbamates. Toxicol Appl Pharmacol. 1973;25(4):569–75.

Rösler M, Anand R, Cicin-Sain A, Gauthier S, Agit Y, Dal-Bianco P, Stähelin HB, Hartman R, Gharabawi M. Efficacy and safety of rivastigmine in patients with Alzheimer's disease: international randomised controlled trial. BMJ. 1999;318(7184):633–8.

Standaert DG, Roberson ED. Treatment of central nervous system degenerative disorders. In: Brunton LL, Chabner BA, Knollmann BC, editors. Goodman & Gil- man's the pharmacologic basis of therapeutics. 12th ed. New York: McGraw-Hill; 2011. p. 609–28.

Case 16
Snake Bite to the Hand

1. Which snakes are venomous in the United States?
2. What is the best field management of rattlesnake envenomations?
3. What are potential effects of rattlesnake venom?
4. What is a dry bite?
5. What laboratory tests should be obtained in all rattlesnake bites?
6. What are indications for administration of antivenom?
7. What are immediate risks associated with antivenom?
8. Are prophylactic antibiotics indicated for rattlesnake envenomations?
9. What are the effects of antivenom?
10. What delayed effects may occur after successful treatment with antivenom?
11. Are blood product transfusions warranted for rattlesnake envenomations?

Abstract Bites from pit vipers (subfamily *Crotalinae*, including rattlesnakes, copperheads, and cottonmouths) comprise the overwhelming majority of venomous snakebites in the United States. Envenomation by these species causes tissue necrosis, edema, and coagulopathy. Rarely, systemic effects including anaphylaxis may also occur. We report a case of a 52-year-old man who sustained a rattlesnake bite to the hand. This case emphasizes the spectrum of clinical effects seen in rattlesnake bites. We describe appropriate treatment including prehospital care, laboratory testing, indications for antivenom administration, criteria for safe discharge, and necessary follow-up.

Keywords Envenomation • Antivenom • Snakebite • Rattlesnake • *Crotalinae* • *Crotalus*

L.R. Dye et al. (eds.), *Case Studies in Medical Toxicology*,
DOI 10.1007/978-3-319-56449-4_16

History of Present Illness

A 52-year-old man presented to the ED 1 h after sustaining a rattlesnake bite to his left 5th digit while working in his garden. He complained of progressive pain to his left hand since the time of envenomation. He denied parasthesias or numbness. He had no chest pain, palpitations, difficulty breathing, wheezing, abdominal pain, nausea, vomiting, diarrhea, or metallic taste.

Which Snakes Are Venomous in the United States?

Pit vipers from the family *Viperidae* (subfamily *Crotalinae*) represent the vast majority of snake envenomations in the United States. Vipers are present in all states except Maine, Alaska, and Hawaii, and envenomations occur most commonly in the warmer months. Pit viper (rattlesnake, copperhead, cottonmouth) venom results in local tissue damage and hematologic toxicity including fibrin degradation and platelet destruction and aggregation.

Coral snakes from the *Elapidae* family are also present in the United States. Elapid venom is neurotoxic, without local tissue effects, and can cause symptoms of parasthesias, weakness, and respiratory muscle paralysis (Gold et al. 2002). In the United States, toxic coral snakes can be differentiated from non-toxic snakes by the approximation of red and yellow color bands, frequently remembered by "red and yellow, kill a fellow."

What Is the Best Field Management of Rattlesnake Envenomations?

Immobilization and elevation of the affected extremity in full extension are important interventions in the prehospital setting (Lavonas et al. 2011a). Pooling of venom in a flexed extremity (i.e., elbow crease) may increase the risk of local soft tissue damage and bleb formation. Alternatively, elevation and extension of the limb will promote lymphatic drainage of venom and may reduce such risk. Patients may require intravenous fluid resuscitation. Anaphylaxis, although rare, should be recognized and treated if present.

Past Medical History	Insulin-dependent diabetes mellitus
	Essential hypertension
Medications	Novolog 30U SQ daily
	Metformin 500 mg PO BID
	Lisinopril 20 mg PO daily
Allergies	NKDA
Family History	Reviewed and non-contributory
Social History	Lives alone. Denies tobacco use, ethanol use, or use of illicit drugs

Physical Examination

Blood pressure	Heart rate	Respiratory rate	Temperature	O_2 saturation
146/84 mmHg	81 bpm	18 breaths/min	37 °C (98.6 °F)	97% (room air)

General: Middle-aged man, no acute distress.
HEENT: Normocephalic, atraumatic, and mucous membranes moist; pupils equal, round, and reactive to light.
Cardiovascular: Regular rate and rhythm, no murmurs.
Pulmonary: lungs clear bilaterally.
Abdomen: Soft, no tenderness to palpation, normal bowel sounds.
Extremities: +tenderness of left axilla, compartments of left upper extremity soft.
Neurologic: Sensation to light touch intact left fifth digit, range of motion of left digits limited by swelling and pain.
Skin: of left upper extremity: Single puncture wound to dorsal aspect of proximal 5th digit with oozing but no purulent discharge; mild warmth and erythema to dorsal ulnar hand and proximal forearm; 3+ edema to dorsal ulnar hand extending to forearm.
Pulses: 2+ equal radial pulses, <2 s capillary refill to distal left 5th digit.

What Are Potential Effects of Rattlesnake Venom?

Rattlesnake venom contains numerous compounds including metalloproteinases, hyaluronidase, and histamine-like factors that cause soft tissue necrosis, inflammation, fluid third spacing, thrombocytopenia, and defibrinating coagulopathy. Rarely, clinically significant and life-threatening bleeding may occur. Hypotension, shock, airway edema, and immune and non-immune anaphylaxis may also occur infrequently (Gold et al. 2002).

What Is a Dry Bite?

A dry bite is one that does not result in venom delivery. Puncture wounds may be seen; however swelling, erythema, significant pain, and bleeding will be absent. In rattlesnakes, dry bites occur in approximately 25% of cases. Dry bites may be difficult to differentiate from true envenomations without serial observation (Lavonas et al. 2011a).

What Laboratory Tests Should Be Obtained in All Rattlesnake Bites?

Complete blood count, prothrombin time (PT) and fibrinogen values should be obtained in all rattlesnake envenomations (Lavonas et al. 2011a). Electrolytes, renal function, and creatinine kinase testing may be useful in selected patients.

Diagnostic Testing

WBC	Hemoglobin	Hematocrit	Platelets
12 k/mm^3	14 g/dL	42%	259 k/mm^3

Na	K	Cl	CO_2	BUN	Cr	Glucose
144 mmol/L	3.5 mmol/L	106 mmol/L	20 mmol/L	23 mg/dL	1.5 mg/dL	110 mg/dL

PT: 10.1 s (reference range: 11.8–14.7 s)
Fibrinogen: 269 mg/dL (reference range: 200–400 mg/dL)

What Are Indications for Administration of Antivenom?

Progressive edema, commonly defined as swelling that extends across one major joint line from the bite site, and coagulation abnormalities (low fibrinogen, low platelets, or elevated PT) are each indications for antivenom. Signs of systemic toxicity including hypotension, nausea, vomiting, and angioedema are also indications for antivenom administration. Each dose of antivenom should be administered over 1 h. More rapid infusions may be used in cases of life-threatening reactions such as hemorrhage or shock (Lavonas et al. 2011b).

What Are Immediate Risks Associated with Antivenom?

Anaphylaxis secondary to antivenom occurs rarely, and serious immediate hypersensitivity reactions are reported in 1.4% of cases. Current, commercially available antivenom is an ovine-derived Fab preparation that is less immunogenic than previous whole IgG formulations. Anaphylaxis secondary to antivenom (or venom) should be treated in a standard fashion with epinephrine, antihistamines, and corticosteroids. Allergy to papaya or sheep is a relative contraindication to antivenom (Cannon et al. 2008).

Are Prophylactic Antibiotics Indicated for Rattlesnake Envenomations?

No. Lymphatic streaking and local tissue damage can be mistaken for cellulitis. However, infection after rattlesnake envenomations is exceedingly rare, reported in approximately 3% of cases. Antibiotics are rarely needed and prophylactic antibiotics are not indicated (LoVecchio et al. 2002).

Initial Treatment

In the ED, the patient was placed in a long arm volar splint, and his extremity was hung in full extension using a stockinette attached to an IV pole. He was given 75 mcg of fentanyl, tetanus booster vaccine, and four vials of Fab antivenom.

Hospital Course

The patient was transferred to a regional toxicology center. On arrival, he complained of progressive pain and swelling to the hand and forearm. Repeat labs showed platelets 276 K/mm^3, PT 15 s, and fibrinogen 128 mg/dL. He was given an additional two vials of antivenom in response to both progressive swelling and lab abnormalities.

Serial circumferential measurements of his hand, forearm, and proximal arm were obtained every 2 h without detection of further swelling. Labs repeated 1 h after the additional antivenom dose showed platelets stable at 273 K/mm^3, PT unchanged at 15 s, and fibrinogen improved but still low at 147 mg/dL. Two additional vials of antivenom were given for persistent coagulopathy and defibrination. Repeat labs 2 h after antivenom showed normalization of PT and fibrinogen at 13 s and 216 mg/dL, respectively.

The patient was observed for 18 h following the last antivenom dose. He had no further progression of swelling and laboratory values remained within normal range. He was discharged home on oral oxycodone/acetaminophen and given follow-up for repeat laboratory draws three and 7 days after envenomation.

What Are the Effects of Antivenom?

Antivenom halts secondary tissue injury, reverses hematologic abnormalities, and reduces systemic venom effects. Antivenom administration has been demonstrated to lower muscular compartment pressures (Gold et al. 2003). Antivenom cannot, however, reverse the local tissue damage that occurs almost immediately upon envenomation (Gutierrez et al. 1998; Homma and Tu 1970).

What Delayed Effects May Occur After Successful Treatment with Antivenom?

The half-life of Fab antivenom is less than that of rattlesnake venom. Due to this discrepancy, delayed recurrence of coagulopathy and thrombocytopenia has been reported in up to 32% of patients (Ruha et al. 2011). Patients treated with antivenom should have follow-up 2–3 days and again 5–7 days after the last antivenom dose to evaluate for recurrence. Delayed serum sickness may rarely occur and typically responds well to treatment with antihistamines and corticosteroids (Cannon et al. 2008).

Are Blood Product Transfusions Warranted for Rattlesnake Envenomations?

In general, blood products are not helpful in treating rattlesnake envenomations. Treatment with antivenom leads to improvement of coagulopathy and thrombocytopenia in almost all patients. For the very rare patients who have had clinically significant bleeding with subsequent anemia, transfusion of red blood cells may be indicated, when given in conjunction with appropriate antivenom therapy and good supportive care (Lavonas et al. 2011a, b).

Specialty-Specific Guidance

Internal Medicine/Family Medicine

- Obtain serial circumferential measurements of the limb at three locations: close to the site of envenomation and on the extremity one and two joints proximal. For example, measure circumferentially around the hand (not including the thumb), the forearm, and the humerus when evaluating a finger envenomation. Marking the exact placement of the measuring tape is helpful for consistency, as is utilization of the same provider in obtaining measurements. This method is thought by experts to be more reliable and reproducible than marking the leading edge of swelling.
- Repeat labs 1 h after completion of each dose of antivenom. Swelling should be monitored as above every 2 h. Repeat doses of antivenom should be given for

increased distal swelling or persistent or new thrombocytopenia, elevation in PT or hypofibrinogenemia. In fact, approximately half of all those envenomated will require additional dosing. With elevation of the extremity, it is expected that the proximal dependent areas of measurement may increase slightly.
- IV opioids may be transitioned to longer acting oral preparations as tolerated. A short course of home oral opioids is frequently required.
- Patients may be discharged home if the exam and laboratory data are stable 18–24 h after the last antivenom dose.
- Any patient receiving antivenom will require follow-up two to three and five to 7 days after last dose of antivenom for evaluation of recurrence.

Prehospital

- Direct attention towards immobilization and elevation of the affected limb.
- Remain vigilant for signs of anaphylaxis including: diffuse erythema, edema, shortness of breath, wheezing, nausea, vomiting, and diarrhea.
- Patients may require fluid resuscitation due to dehydration from outdoor activity or intravascular volume depletion from third spacing.

Emergency Medicine

- Immobilize and elevate the affected limb. For upper extremity envenomations, a long arm volar splint is helpful to assist with immobilization of the elbow and wrist. Hanging the splinted arm from an IV pole is an easy way to achieve sufficient elevation and extension.
- Update tetanus when appropriate.
- Administer intravenous opioid analgesics when needed. Fentanyl is the preferred initial agent in the acute setting owing to minimal histamine release associated with its use. NSAIDs are typically avoided due to potential increased risk of bleeding and platelet dysfunction in these patients.
- Include assessment for distal pulses, proximal (axillary or inguinal) lymph node tenderness, and an extremity neurologic and skin assessment in the physical examination.
- Evaluate for evidence of anaphylaxis or systemic venom effects.
- Obtain a CBC, PT, and fibrinogen in addition to labs otherwise appropriate.
- When indicated (see above), four to six vials of antivenom are typically used as an initial dose for both children and adults. Although rare, patients should be monitored for anaphylaxis during infusion of antivenom.
- Disposition should be to a monitored setting such as the intensive care unit due to risk of anaphylaxis and need for frequent assessment.

- Suspected upper extremity dry bites should be observed for at least 8 h.
- Lower extremity and pediatric envenomations may have delayed presentations. Extended observation periods are often recommended.
- Medical toxicology consultation should be sought before discharging a suspected "dry" bite or any pediatric envenomation.

Critical Care Medicine

- Patients with rattlesnake envenomations may become critically ill. Poison center data reports 1 death per 736 bites. Life-threatening events may include hypotension, hemorrhage, and airway edema.
- Those previously exposed to rattlesnake venom may develop true anaphylaxis after subsequent envenomation.
- Experts consider bites to the head and neck to be high risk for loss of airway and practitioners should have a low threshold for prophylactic intubation.
- Clinically significant, life-threatening bleeding can occur infrequently and may include intracranial hemorrhage or gastrointestinal bleeding. Hemorrhage should be treated with antivenom in addition to blood products when otherwise indicated.
- Venom causes significant swelling and myonecrosis that can be mistaken for compartment syndrome. Compartment syndrome is very rare after rattlesnake envenomations. In most cases, fangs penetrate only into the subcutaneous tissues, not reaching the deeper muscle compartments.
- Antivenom is the treatment of choice in these cases and surgical intervention is rarely required. Patients do, however, frequently develop hemorrhagic blebs at the site of envenomations that may be opened for symptomatic relief.

References

Cannon R, Ruha AM, Kashani J. Acute hypersensitivity reactions associated with administration of crotalidae polyvalent immune Fab antivenom. Ann Emerg Med. 2008;51:407–11.

Gold BS, Dart RC, Barish RA. Bites of venomous snakes. N Engl J Med. 2002;347(5):347–56.

Gold BS, Barish RA, Dart RC, Silverman RP. Resolution of compartment syndrome after rattlesnake envenomation using non-invasive measures. J Emerg Med. 2003;24(3):285–8.

Gutierrez JM, Leon G, Rojas G, Lomonte B. Neutralization of local tissue damage induced by *Bothrops asper* (terciopelo) snake venom. Toxicon. 1998;36(11):1529–38.

Homma M, Tu AT. Antivenin for the treatment of local tissue damage due to envenomation by Southeast Asian snakes. Am J Trop Med Hyg. 1970;19(5):880–4.

Lavonas EJ, Ruha AM, Banner W, Bebarta V. Unified treatment algorithm for the management of crotaline snakebite in the United States: results of an evidence-informed consensus workshop. BMC Emerg Med. 2011a;11:2.

Lavonas EJ, Kokko J, Schaeffer TH, Mlynarchek SL. Short-term outcomes after Fab antivenom therapy for severe crotaline snakebite. Ann Emerg Med. 2011b;57(2):128–37.

LoVecchio F, Klemens J, Welch S, Rodriguez R. Antibiotics after rattlesnake envenomation. J Emerg Med. 2002;23(4):327–8.

Ruha AM, Curry SC, Albrecht C, Riley B. Late hematologic toxicity following treatment of rattlesnake envenomation with crotalidae polyvalent immune Fab antivenom. Toxicon. 2011;57:53–9.

Case 17
Ultra-Rapid Opioid Detoxification

1. What is the differential diagnosis for this patient's altered mental status and pulmonary edema?
2. What is ultra-rapid opioid detox and how is it performed?
3. What are side effects of UROD and ROD?
4. What is the difference between naloxone and naltrexone?
5. What other medications, supplements, or herbal products have been used or reported as treatments for opioid addiction or withdrawal symptoms?
6. Why would someone be exposed to carbon monoxide when undergoing anesthesia?
7. What is spongiform leukencephalopathy?
8. What is ibogaine?

Abstract A 30-year-old male presented to the emergency department after undergoing ultra-rapid opioid detoxification. He was awake but nonverbal for the 8 h following the procedure. With this case, the process of and possible complications associated with ultra-rapid opioid detoxification are reviewed. Potential causes of the patient's symptoms are reviewed, including carbon monoxide poisoning, ibogaine exposure, and spongiform leukencephalopathy.

Keywords Opioid • Ultra-rapid opioid detoxification • Carbon monoxide poisoning • Spongiform leukencephalopathy • Ibogaine

L.R. Dye et al. (eds.), *Case Studies in Medical Toxicology*,
DOI 10.1007/978-3-319-56449-4_17

History of Present Illness

A 30-year-old male was brought from a local detox center, where he underwent ultra-rapid opioid detoxification (UROD), to the emergency department for evaluation of altered mental status. There were no complications reported with this procedure, and the patient was extubated after the procedure without issue. Following extubation, he was awake but had no spontaneous movement and was nonverbal for 8 h prior to transfer to the hospital. During the course of the UROD, patient received propofol, midazolam, cisatracurium, isoflurane, and naloxone (80 mg total). After the procedure, he received an oral dose of naltrexone (100 mg).

Past Medical History	None
Medications	None
Allergies	NKDA
Social History	Substance abuse of opioids. His method of drug use was unknown, but by a friend's report he used oxycodone (900 mg/week) and hydrocodone/acetaminophen tables (100 mg/week).

Physical Examination

Blood pressure	Heart rate	Respiratory rate	Temperature	O_2 saturation
116/65 mmHg	70–85 bpm	42–45 breaths/min	38 °C (100.4 °F)	95% (high flow O_2)

General: Patient was lying on stretcher and had no spontaneous movements.
HEENT: Pupils were 4 mm and reactive. Oropharynx was clear.
Cardiac: Normal rate with no murmurs, gallops, or rubs appreciated.
Pulmonary: Coarse breath sounds present bilaterally throughout both lung fields.
Abdomen: Soft, non-tender, non-distended with active bowel sounds.
Neurologic: Awake and would look at physician when name called. He had normal muscle tone and will withdraw to pain. He has no clonus and mild hyperreflexia. He has minimal spontaneous movements.
Skin: Clear, no abrasions, ecchymosis, or signs of IV drug abuse.

Diagnositic Testing

WBC	Hemoglobin	Platelets
16.9 k/mm^3	16 g/dL	254 k/mm^3

Na	K	Cl	CO_2	BUN/Cr	Glucose
142 mEq/L	3.4 mEq/L	101 mEq/L	26 mEq/L	12/0.6 mg/dL	173 mg/dL

Calcium: 9.3 mg/dL
Magnesium: 1.9 mEq/L
Troponin negative
Venous Blood Gas: pH 7.5; pCO2 34.7; pO2 33; Bicarb 27.3 mmol/L, Oxygen saturation 21%
Lactate: 3.1 mmol/L
Liver function tests (AST, ALT, AP, T bili, albumin): normal
Urinalysis: negative
D-dimer: 353 (normal <200)
Carbon monoxide 1%

Ancillary Testing

CXR: pulmonary congestion; no infiltrate/effusion noted
CT head without contrast: normal

Hospital Course

The patient was admitted to the medical ICU where he developed increasing respiratory distress and pulmonary edema. He was intubated and had normal brain MRI. A CT angiogram for PE was negative and an EEG demonstrated no seizure activity.

What Is the Differential Diagnosis for This patient's Altered Mental Status and Pulmonary Edema?

- Carbon monoxide poisoning from anesthesia
- Medication effect from UROD
- Endocarditis
- Spongiform leukencephalopathy
- Pulmonary embolism
- Partial complex status epilepticus
- Flash pulmonary edema from UROD
- Side effect from attempt at self-detoxification prior to UROD
- Ibogaine toxicity

What Is Ultra-Rapid Opioid Detox and How Is It Performed?

- Ultra-rapid opioid detox (UROD) or anesthesia-assisted rapid opioid detoxification (AAROD) and rapid opioid detox (ROD) are rapid detoxification methods provided to patients with heroin and opioid dependency. There are no uniform protocols and the goal is to minimize perceived withdrawal symptoms through anesthesia or sedation. General principles for this procedure include use of alpha-2 agonist, anesthetic or sedation, and opioid-antagonist. High doses of opioid-antagonists are used.

ROD	UROD
Sedation	General anesthesia
Naloxone	Naloxone
Naltrexone	Naltrexone
Duration 6–72 h	Duration <6 h (usually 4–5 h)

- Occasionally, patients are discharged on clonidine or with naltrexone tablets placed under the skin.
- UROD and ROD are not supported by any professional organizations due to concerns about the safety of the procedures and no proven benefit of UROD or ROD. There are higher adverse effects in patients undergoing UROD/ROD when compared to inpatient opioid withdrawal with clonidine or buprenorphine. Additionally, there is no difference in relapse rate for heroin use at 6 months. (American Society of Addiction Medicine 2005; Karan and Martin 2011; WHO 2009)

What Are Side Effects of UROD and ROD?

- Minor residual withdrawal effects including anxiety, restlessness, and yawning are reported after completion of this procedure (Safari et al. 2010).
- As evidenced by this case, massive pulmonary edema can occur in the setting of UROD. There are multiple case reports of pulmonary edema associated with UROD (Berlin et al. 2013). It is unclear from the literature if this is a direct effect of the naloxone or from the opioid, as this has also been reported with routine naloxone use for reversal of opioid intoxication and opioid intoxication (Steinberg and Karliner 1968; Gopinathan et al. 1970; Frand et al. 1972; Flacke et al. 1977; Taff 1983; Partridge and Ward 1986; Prough et al. 1984)
- Nausea, vomiting, and diarrhea (Berlin et al. 2013)
- Hypokalemia (Berlin et al. 2013)
- Cerebral edema (Berlin et al. 2013)
- Cardiac arrest while undergoing procedure (Berlin et al. 2013)
- Accidental overdose when relapsing and using pre-UROD/ROD amounts of drugs (Salami et al. 2014)

What Is the Difference Between Naloxone and Naltrexone?

- Naloxone is frequently used to reverse opioid toxicity, whereas naltrexone is used to maintain abstinence once opioids are out of a patient's system.
- Naloxone has poor oral bioavailability, but can be used orally to treat opioid-related constipation. For treatment of opioid toxicity, naloxone is typically given intravenously, intramuscularly, or intranasally.
- Oral naltrexone is rapidly absorbed and has a long duration of action (half-life of approximately 72 h) (Lee et al. 1988). It is also available in a sustained release intramuscular form for monthly dosing.
- Naltrexone has also been used to treat alcoholism (Kranzler and Modesto-Lowe 1998)

What Other Medications, Supplements, or Herbal Products Have Been Used or Reported as Treatments for Opioid Addiction or Withdrawal Symptoms?

While many medications, supplements, and herbal products have been used in the treatment of opioid addiction and for withdrawal symptoms, not all are efficacious and many have not formally been evaluated for this process.

- Medications used primarily as treatment for opioid addiction:
  - Methadone
  - Buprenorphine (available as tablet, transdermal patch, intramuscular depot version, sublingual film)
  - Slow-release morphine
  - Dihydrocodeine
  - Tramadol
  - Naltrexone (available as a tablet and intramuscular depot injection)
  - Kratom (*Mitragynia speciosa korth*)
- Products used primarily to treat withdrawal symptoms:
  - Clonidine
  - Diphenoxylate/atropine
  - Antiemetics
  - Diphenhydramine
  - Acetaminophen, ibuprofen, or products in combination with diphenhydramine to help with sleeping at night
  - Nicotinamide
  - Kratom (*Mitragynia speciosa korth*)

Why Would Someone Be Exposed to Carbon Monoxide When Undergoing Anesthesia?

- There have been previous case reports of carbon monoxide toxicity developing in patients receiving anesthesia. These patients were often undergoing procedures on Mondays or Tuesdays in operating rooms that had been idle for >24 h (Firth and Stuckey 1945; Middleton et al. 1965; Pearson et al. 2001).
- The proposed mechanism for the exposure to CO was interaction between the anesthetic gases and CO2 absorbent granules, which resulted in CO production (Moon et al. 1991; Pearson et al. 2001).
- CO production in anesthesia units is determined by four primary elements—the type of CO2 granule in the anesthesia circuit, the temperature of the room, type of anesthesia used, and the "dryness" of the granules (Fang et al. 1995).

What Is Spongiform Leukencephalopathy?

- Spongiform leukencephalopathy is a progressive neurologic disorder. (Kriegstein et al. 1997; Rizzuto et al. 1997)
- It involves diffuse spongiform demyelination of the white matter, also called vacuolating myelinopathy, which is related to inhaling heroin fumes by "chasing the dragon" (inhalation of fumes created when heroin powder is heated on a piece of foil).
- Associated symptoms include ataxia, dysarthria, mutism, muscle spasticity, dysmetria, hyperreflexia (Sempere et al. 1991; Kriegstein et al. 1999; Celius and Andersson 1996; Buttner et al. 2000)

What Is Ibogaine?

- A schedule I, hallucinogenic alkaloid found in an African shrub *Tabernanthe iboga*.
- It has been used for opioid detoxification/ease the symptoms of withdrawal although it is not approved for this (Alper et al. 2000)
- Serious side effects such as prolonged QT interval, polymorphic ventricular tachycardia, and death have been reported following ibogaine use, but it is unknown if this was truly a direct effect of ibogaine or result of the combination of ibogaine with underlying comorbidities (Asua 2013; Alper et al. 2012)

Case Conclusion

In this case, the patient underwent ultra-rapid opioid detoxification and developed pulmonary edema. UROD is not recommended or approved for opioid detoxification, but many people seek this treatment as an alternative for opioid detoxification. This patient developed pulmonary edema, a complication of rapid opioid reversal that is also seen with naloxone administration. Supportive care with intubation was required, but the patient did well, was extubated, and discharged home on hospital day two.

Specialty-Specific Guidance

Internal Medicine/Family Medicine

- ROD/UROD is not supported by any professional organizations due to safety issues.
- Medical insurance does not cover expenses related to ROD/UROD.
- Candid discussions with patients regarding safer detoxification programs should be undertaken if patients are looking for a detoxification program or are struggling with opiate/opioid addiction.

Emergency Medicine

- Obtaining as much information as possible from the anesthesiologist who performed the procedure is necessary for all patients who undergo ROD/UROD. Additionally, obtaining a list of medications and information about any noted complication during the ROD/UROD is very important.
- Information provided by accompanying friends/family can also be very helpful.
- Consider broad differential diagnoses, including infectious etiology, for all patients presenting after ROD/UROD.
- Any implanted opioid-antagonist needs to be removed in patients experiencing complications from this type of procedure.
- Respiratory distress may be an early sign of underlying pulmonary edema and should be managed with CPAP or endotracheal intubation.
- Consult your regional poison control center or medical toxicology service for guidance in patient treatment and when entertaining other diagnoses.

Toxicology

- Obtaining as much information as possible from the anesthesiologist who performed the procedure is necessary for all patients who undergo ROD/UROD. Additionally, obtaining a list of medications and information about any noted complication during the ROD/UROD is very important.
- Information provided by accompanying friends/family can also be very helpful.
- Consider broad differential diagnoses, including infectious etiology, for all patients presenting after ROD/UROD.
- Any implanted opioid-antagonist needs to be removed in patients experiencing complications from this type of procedure.
- Respiratory distress may be an early sign of underlying pulmonary edema and should be managed with CPAP or endotracheal intubation.
- Co-exposure of other potential opioid detoxification medication/supplements should be considered.

References

Alper KR, Lotsof HS, Frenken GM, Luciano DJ, Bastiaans J. Ibogaine in acute opioid withdrawal: an open label case series. Ann N Y Acad Sci. 2000;909:257–9.

Alper KR, Stajic M, Gill JR. Fatalities temporally associated with the ingestion of ibogaine. J Forensic Sci. 2012;57(2):398–412.

American Society of Addiction Medicine. Public policy state on rapid and ultra-rapid opioid detoxification. 2005; Available via American Society of Addiction Medicine: http://www.asam.org/advocacy/find-a-policy-statement/view-policy-statement/public-policy-statements/2011/12/15/rapid-and-ultra-rapid-opioid-detoxification. Accessed 18 Jan 2015.

Asua I. Growing menace of ibogaine toxicity. Br J Anaesth. 2013;111(6):1029–30.

Berlin D, Farmer BM, Rao RB, et al. Deaths and severe adverse events associated with anesthesia-assisted rapid opioid detoxification. MMWR. 2013;62(38):777–80.

Buttner A, Mall G, Penning R, Weis S. The neuropathology of heroin abuse. Forensic Sci Int. 2000;113(1–3):435–42.

Celius EG, Andersson S. Leucoencephalopathy after inhalation of heroin: a case report. J Neurol Neurosurg Psychiatry. 1996;60:694–5.

Fang ZX, Eger EI, Laster MJ, Chortkoff BS, Kandel L, Ionescu P. Carbon monoxide production from degradation of desflurane, enflurane, isoflurane, halothane, and sevoflurane by soda lime and Baralyme. Anesth Analg. 1995;80:1187–93.

Firth JB, Stuckey RE. Decomposition of trichloroethylene in closed circuit anesthesia. Lancet. 1945;1:814–6.

Flacke JW, Flacke WE, Williams GD. Acute pulmonary edema following naloxone reversal of high-dose morphine anesthesia. Anesthesiology. 1977;47:376–8.

Frand UI, Shim CS, Williams MH. Methadone-induced pulmonary edema. Ann Intern Med. 1972;76:975–9.

Gopinathan K, Saroj D, Spears J, et al. Hemodynamic studies in heroin induced acute pulmonary edema. Circulation. 1970;42:44.

Karan L, Martin J. Anesthesia-assisted rapid opioid detoxification. Available via: California Society of Addiction Medicine. 2011. http://www.csam-asam.org/anesthesia-assisted-rapidopioid-detoxification. Accessed 14 Jan 2015.

Kranzler H, Modesto-Lowe V, Nuwayser ES. Sustained-release naltrexone for alcoholism treatment: a preliminary study. Alcohol Clin Exp Res. 1998;22(5):1074–9.
Kriegstein AR, Armitage BA, Kim PY. Heroin inhalation and progressive spongiform leukencephalopathy. NEJM. 1997;336(8):589–90.
Kriegstein AR, Sungu DC, Millar WS, et al. Leukencephalopathy and raised brain lactate from heroin vapor inhalation ("chasing the dragon"). Neurology. 1999;53(8):1765–73.
Lee M, Wagner H, Tanada S, Frost J, Bice A, Dannals R. Duration of occupancy of opiate receptors by naltrexone. J Nucl Med. 1988;29:1207–11.
Middleton V, vanPoznak A, Artusio JF Jr, Smith SM. Carbon monoxide accumulation in closed circuit anesthesia systems. Anesthesiology. 1965;26:715–0.
Moon R, Ingram C, Brunner E, Meyer A. Spontaneous generation of carbon monoxide within anesthesia circuits. Anesthesiology. 1991;75:A873.
Partridge BL, Ward CF. Pulmonary edema following low-dose naloxone administration. Anesthesiology. 1986;65:709–10.
Pearson ML, Levine WC, Finton RJ, et al. Anesthesia-associated carbon monoxide exposure among surgical patients. Infect Control Hosp Epidemiol. 2001;22(6):352–6.
Prough DS, Roy R, Bumgarner J, et al. Acute pulmonary edema in healthy teenagers following conservative doses of intravenous naloxone. Anesthesiology. 1984;60:485–6.
Rizzuto N, Morbin M, Ferrari S, et al. Delayed spongiform leukencephalopathy after heroin abuse. Acta Neuropathol. 1997;94:87–90.
Safari F, Mottaghi K, Malek S, Salimi A. Effect of ultra-rapid opiate detoxification on withdrawal syndrome. J Addict Dis. 2010;29(4):449–54.
Salami A, Safari F, Mohajerani SA, et al. Long-term relapse of ultra-rapid opioid detoxification. J Addict Dis. 2014;33:33–40.
Sempere AP, Posada I, Ramo C, Cabello A. Spongiform leucoencephalopathy after inhaling heroin. Lancet. 1991;338:320.
Steinberg AD, Karliner JS. The clinical spectrum of heroin pulmonary edema. Arch Intern Med. 1968;122:122–7.
Taff RH. Pulmonary edema following naloxone administration in a patient without heart disease. Anesthesiology. 1983;59:576–7.
World Health Organization. Guidelines for the psychosocially assisted pharmacological treatment of opioid dependence. Geneva, Switzerland. 2009. http://apps.who.int/iris/handle/10665/43948. Accessed 22 Feb 2016.

Case 18
Concentrated Hydrogen Peroxide Ingestion

1. What are the toxic effects of concentrated hydrogen peroxide?
2. What diagnostic workup is required after concentrated H_2O_2 ingestion?
3. What is the management of toxic pneumobilia?

Abstract A 32-year-old man ingests concentrated hydrogen peroxide and develops vomiting and abdominal pain. The diagnostic workup and management approach is discussed, including the role of imaging and hyperbaric oxygen therapy.

Keywords Hydrogen peroxide • Caustics • Gas embolism • Hyperbaric oxygen

History of Present Illness

A previously healthy 32-year-old man presented to the ED after unintentionally ingesting a mouthful of 35% hydrogen peroxide (H_2O_2) from an unmarked bottle he kept in his refrigerator. He was using the solution to clean produce. Upon realizing his error, he immediately drank a liter of water, which promptly induced vomiting. In the ED, the patient complained of mild throat and chest discomfort as well as "abdominal fullness."

Past Medical History	None
Medications	None
Allergies	None
Social History	Denied alcohol, smoking, or illicit drug use

L.R. Dye et al. (eds.), *Case Studies in Medical Toxicology*,
DOI 10.1007/978-3-319-56449-4_18

Physical Examination

Blood pressure	Heart rate	Respiratory rate	Temperature	O_2 saturation
140/92 bpm	93 bpm	18 breaths/min	35.8 ° C (96.4 °F)	98%

General: Comfortable, nontoxic appearing.
HEENT: Voice normal, normal lips, and oropharynx.
Cardiovascular: Regular rate and rhythm.
Pulmonary: Symmetric breath sounds, clear to auscultation.
Abdomen: Scaphoid abdomen, tender epigastrium.
Neurologic: Alert and oriented to person, place, and time.
Skin: Warm and well-perfused.

Ancillary Testing

Abdominal x-ray: normal, no portal venous air detected.
CT abdomen: extensive air throughout the portal venous system.

Hospital Course

Hyperbaric oxygen therapy was recommended for the patient in this case, but transfer to a hyperbaric facility was not possible. He was instead admitted to the hospital for continuous monitoring. Over the next 12 h, his symptoms gradually resolved, and a repeat CT scan the following day showed complete resolution of the portal venous gas. The patient was subsequently discharged without any sequelae.

Key Points of Case

What Are Potential Exposures to Hydrogen Peroxide?

H_2O_2 is a colorless and odorless liquid. Solutions with concentrations ranging from 3% to 5% have many household applications, including use as a wound disinfectant and dentifrice; dilute solutions are also utilized for similar purposes in the hospital setting. Industrial-strength H_2O_2 (concentrations of 10–35%) is employed to bleach textiles and paper, and higher concentrations (70–90%) are used as an oxygen source for rocket engines.

Consumer application of concentrated H_2O_2 solutions has become increasingly common. Some, like this patient, clean the surfaces of fruits and vegetables with

H_2O_2 to decrease transmission of bacteria during cutting (Ukuku et al. 2005). More concerning, however, is the purported medicinal benefits of ingesting "food grade" (35%) H_2O_2 mixed with water—touted on many Internet sites as a treatment for illnesses such as emphysema, cancer, anemia, and HIV (theoneminutemiracle.com). Sometimes referred to as "hyperoxygenation therapy," this so-called treatment has not been approved by the US Food and Drug Administration for any such purpose (FDA news release 2006). When diluted sufficiently, this concoction is not harmful, but unlikely to provide any health benefits.

What Are the Toxic Effects of Concentrated Hydrogen Peroxide?

Injury from concentrated H_2O_2 consumption is primarily from either direct caustic injury or the embolic obstruction of blood flow. Following ingestion, the enzyme catalase metabolizes the breakdown of H_2O_2 in accordance with the following equation: $2H_2O_2(aq) \rightarrow 2H_2O(l) + O_2(g) + \text{heat}$. A single milliliter (mL) of 35% H_2O_2 results in the liberation of 100 mL of O_2. (The more common 3% household solution generates 10 mL of oxygen per 1 mL of H_2O_2.) The creation of a large intragastric pressure gradient from the liberation of gas, coupled with the caustic and exothermic injury of the bowel mucosa, may contribute to the movement of oxygen through epithelial interstices into the circulation. In addition, and perhaps more importantly, absorption of intact H_2O_2 with subsequent metabolism by catalase in the blood liberates oxygen directly within the vasculature. Oxygen bubbles may coalesce in blood circulation and occlude vascular flow. In canine studies, elevated oxygen tension in the portal venous system led to cessation of mesenteric flow in arteries and veins, though the mechanism of action is unclear (Shaw et al. 1967). Furthermore, coalescence of bubbles can lead to disruption of bowel-cell architecture, fibrin plugging of capillaries, venous thrombosis, and infarction of tissues (Shaw et al. 1967).

Cases of cardiac and cerebral gas embolism have been reported and present similarly to patients with diving-related decompression injuries (e.g., stroke-like syndromes) (Cina et al. 1994; Rider et al. 2008). The proposed mechanism for these latter effects involves the metabolism of H_2O_2 in the systemic circulation with production of oxygen bubbles. In the presence of a septal defect, bubbles may move from the right heart to the arterial circulation (French et al. 2010).

Toxicity and death from H_2O_2 exposure associated with the historical treatment of inspissated meconium (Shaw et al. 1967) as well as the irrigation of wounds (Bassan et al. 1982) has been reported. Ingestion of a 3% solution is generally benign, resulting at worst in gastrointestinal symptoms or throat irritation (Henry et al. 1996). Rarely does significant toxicity occur at this low concentration (Cina et al. 1994) with the vast majority of such cases involving concentrated solutions of 35%.

What Diagnostic Workup Is Required After Concentrated H_2O_2 Ingestion?

Reportedly, ingestion of as little as a "sip" or "mouthful" of 35% H_2O_2 has resulted in venous and arterial gas embolism, occasionally with severe consequences, but no current consensus guidelines exist regarding imaging requirements (Rider et al. 2008). Some toxicologists and hyperbaric physicians believe that the presence of portal venous air does not adversely impact a patient's prognosis or necessitate treatment, and therefore, a workup is unnecessary. Others, however, suggest that the presence of portal venous air indicates oversaturation of oxygen in the blood, placing the patient at increased risk for cardiac and cerebral air embolism. Although practice patterns vary by institution, it is reasonable that patients presenting with abdominal complaints after ingestion of H_2O_2 undergo imaging to assess for portal venous air. The presence of portal venous air may often be identified on X-ray imaging (Rackoff and Merton 1990; Luu et al. 1992); however, it lacks sensitivity (Burns and Schmidt 2013), as was the case in our patient. Therefore, if X-ray is normal, it is reasonable to obtain CT imaging to assess for portal venous air.

Concentrated H_2O_2 ingestions may be associated with significant gastritis and mucosal injury. Endoscopy is recommended within 12–24 h of ingestion to assess degree of injury in all patients with intentional ingestions, and in patients with unintentional ingestions and presence of stridor, or having two of three symptoms of: vomiting, abdominal pain, or drooling (Fulton 2011).

Toxic Pneumobilia: Management?

The management of patients with portal venous gas following H_2O_2 ingestion is controversial and has not been established. Microbubble formation in the vasculature may lead to platelet aggregation and release of platelet activator inhibitor (Mirski et al. 2007), a mechanism that may theoretically respond to administration of a platelet inhibitor, such as aspirin, in these patients. Hyperbaric oxygen therapy involves increasing the ambient pressure by several atmospheres inside a specially designed chamber—the same therapy used for diving-related decompression injury. Hyperbaric oxygen therapy increases the amount of dissolved oxygen in the blood, thereby decreasing bubble formation and allowing transport of dissolved oxygen to the lungs where it can be exhaled. Some patients with portal venous air experience significant pain and portal venous hypertension, which may respond rapidly to this therapy (Papafragkou et al. 2012). Based on available literature, hyperbaric therapy is reasonable for patients with significant abdominal pain and portal venous air following H_2O_2 ingestion; less controversial is the role of hyperbaric therapy in those with cerebral air embolism. Multiple case reports of patients with significant neurologic findings demonstrate resolution of symptoms following hyperbaric therapy (Rider et al. 2008).

Specialty-Specific Guidance

Emergency Medicine

- Ingestion of household concentration H_2O_2 (3–5%) may result in mild gastric irritation and is typically well-tolerated
- Ingestion of concentrated, "food grade" H_2O_2 (35%) may cause significant caustic injury and can result in venous and arterial gas embolism

Patients Who Have Ingested 35% H_2O_2

- Symptoms associated with ingestion includes:
  - Gastrointestinal

    Nausea, vomiting
    Abdominal pain
    Oropharyngeal irritation

  - Neurologic (related to cerebral gas embolism)

    Drowsiness, lethargy, coma
    Stroke-like symptoms (cranial nerve deficits, hemiparesis, hemiplegia, sensory deficits, ataxia, dysarthria)

- Diagnostic imaging:
  - Abdominal X-ray is indicated to assess for the presence of portal venous air in patients with significant abdominal pain
  - CT abdomen should be considered in patients with negative abdominal X-ray
  - CT head is indicated for all patients with neurologic symptoms
- Management
  - Esophagogastroduodenoscopy should be considered to assess for caustic injury
  - Use of hyperbaric oxygen therapy is controversial, but is reasonable to consider in:

    Any patients with CT evidence of cerebral embolism or in patients with stroke-like symptoms where concern exists for cerebral gas embolism
    Select patients with significant abdominal pain and portal venous air present on CT imaging

References

35% H_2O_2 hydrogen peroxide food grade certified benefits. 2015. http://www.theoneminutemiracleinc.com/pages/h2o2-benefits/.

Bassan MM, Dudai M, Shalev O. Near-fatal systemic oxygen embolism due to wound irrigation with hydrogen peroxide. Postgrad Med J. 1982;58(681):448–50.

Burns RA, Schmidt SM. Portal venous gas emboli after accidental ingestion of concentrated hydrogen peroxide. J Emerg Med. 2013;45(3):345–7.

Cina SJ, Downs JC, Conradi SE. Hydrogen peroxide: a source of lethal oxygen embolism. Case report and review of the literature. Am J Forensic Med Pathol. 1994;15(1):44–50.

FDA warns consumers against drinking high-strength hydrogen peroxide for medicinal use: ingestion can lead to serious health risk and death [news release]. Silver Spring, MD: US Food and Drug Administration. 2006. http://www.fda.gov/NewsEvents/Newsroom/PressAnnouncements/2006/ucm108701.htm. [30 January 2015].

French LK, Horowitz BZ, McKeown NJ. Hydrogen peroxide ingestion associated with portal venous gas and treatment with hyperbaric oxygen: a case series and review of the literature. Clin Toxicol (Phila). 2010;48(6):533–8.

Fulton JA. Caustics. In: Nelson LS, Lewin NA, Howland MA, Hoffman RS, Goldfrank LR, Flomenbaum NE, editors. Goldfrank's toxicological emergencies. 9th ed. New York: McGraw-Hill; 2011. p. 1364–73.

Henry MC, Wheeler J, Mofenson HC, et al. Hydrogen peroxide 3% exposures. J Toxicol Clin Toxicol. 1996;34(3):323–7.

Luu TA, Kelley MT, Strauch JA, Avradopoulos K. Portal vein gas embolism from hydrogen peroxide ingestion. Ann Emerg Med. 1992;21(11):1391–3.

Mirski MA, Lele AV, Fitzsimmons L, Toung TJK. Diagnosis and treatment of vascular air embolism. Anesthesiology. 2007;106:164–77.

Papafragkou S, Gasparyan A, Batista R, Scott P. Treatment of portal venous gas embolism with hyperbaric oxygen after accidental ingestion of hydrogen peroxide: a case report and review of the literature. J Emerg Med. 2012;43(1):e21–3.

Rackoff WR, Merton DF. Gas embolism after ingestion of hydrogen peroxide. Pediatrics. 1990;85(4):593–4.

Rider SP, Jackson SB, Rusyniak DE. Cerebral air gas embolism from concentrated hydrogen peroxide ingestion. Clin Toxicol (Phila). 2008;46(9):815–8.

Shaw A, Cooperman A, Fusco J. Gas embolism produced by hydrogen peroxide. N Engl J Med. 1967;277(5):238–41.

Ukuku DO, Bari ML, Kawamoto S, Isshiki K. Use of hydrogen peroxide in combination with nisin, sodium lactate and citric acid for reducing transfer of bacterial pathogens from whole melon surfaces to fresh-cut pieces. Int J Food Microbiol. 2005;104(2):225–33.

Case 19
Nicotine Toxicity

1. What is your differential diagnosis?
2. Why is isopropanol on the differential?
3. What are the symptoms of GHB toxicity?
4. What is GHB used for?
5. What are the symptoms of nicotine toxicity?
6. What are other sources of nicotine?
7. What are the basics for management?
8. How much nicotine is too much?
9. How does one determine if a patient with an exposure is going to get sick?
10. What are some of the most common effects seen in adults who attempt suicide with nicotine patches?
11. How do electronic cigarettes work?
12. Does the FDA regulate electronic cigarettes?
13. How many different brands of electronic cigarettes are available to purchase? How many flavors?
14. What plant has been used as a smoking cessation medication in Eastern Europe and can cause nicotine-like effects with exposure?
15. What other plants can have nicotine-like effects?

Abstract In this chapter, we discuss the case of a toddler who acutely vomited following ingestion of a small container of liquid on his father's nightstand. He subsequently developed ataxia and lethargy. This chapter explores possible causes of his symptoms, including GHB intoxication and nicotine exposure.

Keywords Seizures • Electronic cigarettes • Nicotine • GHB

L.R. Dye et al. (eds.), *Case Studies in Medical Toxicology*,
DOI 10.1007/978-3-319-56449-4_19

History of Present Illness

- A 2-year-old male was brought to emergency department by his father for evaluation after developing several episodes of emesis following an ingestion of about 2 mL liquid from small container on father's nightstand.
- The patient rapidly became lethargic and ataxic when attempting to stand after being brought back from the triage area.

Past Medical History	None
Medications	None
Allergies	NKDA
Social History	Lives at home with parents; no smoking in the home

Physical Examination

Blood pressure	Heart rate	Respiratory rate	Temperature	O_2 saturation
109/69 mmHg	160 bpm	24 breaths/min	36.9 °C (98.5 °F)	100% (room air)

General: The patient was pale and diaphoretic.
HEENT: Pupils were midsize and reactive, no nystagmus.
Cardiovascular: Tachycardia but no M/R/G. Distal pulses present bilaterally in all extremities.
Pulmonary: Chest was clear to auscultation bilaterally with no wheezes, rales, or rhonchi. There was no accessory muscle use or stridor noted.
Abdomen: Hyperactive bowel sounds, but abdomen soft and non-tender. Patient continued to vomit non-bloody, non-bilious emesis in the ED.
Neurologic: Generalized weakness, unsteady gait, lethargy but no tremor noted.

What Is Your Differential Diagnosis?

- Ipecac ingestion
- Ethanol ingestion
- Isopropanol ingestion or dermal exposure
- Gamma-hydroxybutyrate (GHB) ingestion
- Ingestion of nicotine liquid replacement for electronic cigarettes

Why Is Isopropanol on the Differential?

Isopropanol is highly inebriating (more so than ethanol) and is an irritant that can cause vomiting.

What Are the Symptoms of GHB Toxicity?

- Patients with GHB intoxication frequently present with bradycardia, hypothermia, hypotension, respiratory depression (Liechti et al. 2006)
- They also can develop CNS depression, salivation, vomiting, myoclonus that can appear seizure-like, and coma (Liechti et al. 2006)
- Deaths are rare from isolated GHB use, but have been reported (Knudsen et al. 2008, 2010).

What Is GHB Used for?

- Medical therapy for narcolepsy (Brown and Guilleminault 2011)
- Treatment of alcohol abuse and withdrawal (Maremmani et al. 2001)
- As an anabolic steroid by body builders (Brennan and Van Hout 2014)
- To facilitate date rape (Brennan and Van Hout 2014)
- Recreational drug abuse (Brennan and Van Hout 2014)

Diagnostic Testing

WBC	Hemoglobin	Platelets
14.1 k/mm^3	9.8/30 g/dL	212 k/mm^3

Na	K	Cl	CO_2	BUN/Cr	Glucose
137 mmol/L	4.2 mmol/L	105 mmol/L	24 mmol/L	14/0.3 mg/dL	128 mg/dL

Calcium: 9.4 mg/dL
LFTS: within normal limits
Ethanol level (serum): negative
Acetaminophen: negative
Salicylic acid: negative

Ancillary Testing

An EKG was performed and demonstrated sinus tachycardia with normal intervals and no signs of acute ischemia.

Hospital Course

Intravenous fluids were started; the patient was placed on a cardiac monitor and observed. No other medications were administered as the child began to improve with decreased episodes of emesis in the emergency department. Additionally, there was some hope that any continued emesis would act as a means of self-decontamination. He was admitted to the hospital for continued observation.

The liquid was identified as an e cigarette refill bottle containing 10 mL of 16–24 mg nicotine.

What Are the Symptoms of Nicotine Toxicity?

Mild toxicity:

- Nausea, vomiting, diarrhea
- Tremors
- Tachycardia, tachypnea, and increased blood pressure

Severe toxicity:

- Biphasic effect with symptoms of cholinergic excess initially (minutes to hours) and bradycardia, coma, neuromuscular blockade, which can result in respiratory failure and hypotension late (few hours) in severe toxicity.
- Can see salivation, diaphoresis, nausea, vomiting and diarrhea within minutes of significant ingestion.
- Other symptoms include dysrhythmias, muscle fasciculations, confusion, ataxia, headache, dizziness, and seizures.
- Vomiting is most common initial symptom; however, the development of seizures without vomiting as the initial symptom following ingestion of liquid nicotine has been reported (Lookabill and Beuhler 2014, pers. comm. 8 September).
- There are multiple cases in the literature of deaths attributed to nicotine ingestions. In one of the reports, the deceased extracted nicotine from tobacco (Corkery et al. 2010). In another report, the patient drank a liquid nicotine preparation, as well as a large amount of alcohol (Solarino et al. 2010). A pediatric death related to the accidental ingestion of liquid nicotine for an electronic cigarette refill has also been reported (Eggleston et al. 2016).

What Are Other Sources of Nicotine?

- Cigarettes (10–30 mg/cigarette)
- Cigarette butts (5–7 mg/butt)
- Nicotine gum (2–4 mg/piece)
- Nicotine lozenges (2–4 mg/lozenge)
- Nicotine patches (8.3–114 mg/patch)
- Nicotine pesticides
- Fresh or dry tobacco leaves
- Tobacco extract and tobacco smoke enemas

What Are the Basics for Treatment Management?

- Ingestions are managed with supportive care primarily.
- Pesticide exposures and dermal exposure patients should be decontaminated with soap and water with providers being careful to wear personal protective equipment.
- Activated charcoal is not recommended, even though it can bind nicotine, due to rapid absorption, associated risk of vomiting, and potential for seizures (potential risk outweighs benefit).

How Much Nicotine Is Too Much?

- In general, the LD50 of nicotine in adults is accepted as 0.5–1 mg/kg; however, a recent paper suggests the LD50 may be much higher at 6.5–13 mg/kg (Kobert 1906; Mayer 2014).
- Based on symptoms of toxicity being noted in children who ingested one cigarette or three cigarette butts, physicians should be concerned for any child <6-year-old who ingests these amounts (Smolskine et al. 1988)
- Severe toxicity has been reported in a single case report of a child who ingested a total of 2 mg of nicotine from a piece of nicotine gum (Mensch and Holden 1984)

How Does One Determine If a Patient with an Exposure Is Going to Get Sick?

- Due to rapid mucosal absorption of some products, ingested gums, lozenges, and chewed patches may produce symptoms within a few minutes. Other ingestions may not produce symptoms up to 90 min. Expected initial symptoms would include vomiting and mild symptoms as noted above.
- Any child with symptoms should be observed until symptom free with normal vital signs.

- Adults with minor symptoms from accidental exposures may not necessarily require medical evaluation, but those who intentionally ingested nicotine containing products or develop vomiting should be observed for development of worsening symptoms. Most reports of ingestions resulting in mild to moderate toxicity and even some with severe toxicity note resolution of symptoms within 12–24 h.
- Patients with dermal exposures from wet/fresh tobacco leaves may not develop symptoms for 3–17 h from the time of exposure and symptoms can last for several days.
- Patients with patch exposures may continue to have nicotine absorption from area where patch (es) were located due to subcutaneous deposition of nicotine (Soghoian 2010).

Hospital Course Continued

The patient was admitted overnight and returned back to baseline by the morning with normal repeat labs and vital signs. He was discharged home on hospital day two.

What Are some of the most Common Effects Seen in Adults Who Attempt Suicide with Nicotine Patches?

- In a case series of adults who intentionally placed excessive nicotine patches as a suicide attempt, the most common findings were dizziness, hypertension, diaphoresis, and altered mental status (Woolf et al. 1996).

How Do Electronic Cigarettes Work?

- When a person takes a drag from an electronic cigarette, it triggers a microprocessor to heat a metal coil in order to vaporize liquid nicotine and that vapor is then inhaled.
- The liquid nicotine is contained in a cartridge that is either fully replaced or can be refilled.
- The nicotine is usually dissolved in vegetable oil or propylene glycol (Caponnetto et al. 2012).

Does the FDA Regulate Electronic Cigarettes?

- In 2016, the FDA extended its regulatory authority to cover all tobacco products, to include electronic cigarettes and electronic liquids, including flavorings. This includes regulation of "manufacturing, importing, packaging, labeling,

advertising, promotions, sales, and distribution of electronic nicotine delivery systems" (FDA 2016).
- Prior to this, the FDA center for Tobacco Products only regulated cigarettes, cigarette tobacco, roll-your-own tobacco, and smokeless tobacco, but not non-tobacco based nicotine products.
- The FDA Center for Drug Evaluation and Research regulates electronic cigarettes specifically marketed for therapeutic purposes (ex: products marketed for smoking cessation).

How Many Different Brands of Electronic Cigarettes Are Available to Purchase? How Many Flavors?

- One recent study found 466 brands of e cigarettes marketed on the internet as of January 2014, with 7764 unique flavors among them.
- The same study group found only 250 brands in 2012. Furthermore, in the 17 months between the searches, there was a net increase of 10.5 brands and 242 new flavors per month (Zhu et al. 2014).

What Plant Has Been Used as a Smoking Cessation Medication in Eastern Europe and Can Cause Nicotine-Like Effects with Exposure?

- Plants from the Leguminsoae family contain cystisine, a nicotinic alkaloid, which works as a partial agonist at the receptor level.
- It was found to be superior to nicotine replacement therapy in a recent clinical trial (Walker et al. 2014).

What Other Plants Can Have Nicotine-Like Effects?

- Plants containing nicotine and nicotine-like alkaloids that have been reported to be poisonous to humans include *Conium maculatum*, *Nicotiana glauca* and *Nicotiana tabacum*, *Laburnum anagyroides*, *Caulophyllum thalictroides*, and *Baptisia*.
- These plants contain the toxic alkaloids nicotine, anabasine, cytisine, *n*-methylcytisine, coniine, *n*-methylconiine, and γ-coniceine. These alkaloids are readily absorbed via dermal and oral routes and have high volumes of distribution.
- Symptoms typically follow a biphasic pattern where initial symptoms are consistent with nicotinic cholinergic poisoning: tremor, tachycardia, hypertension, abdominal pain followed by a period of hypotension, bradycardia, respiratory distress, and coma (Schep et al. 2009; Anderson 2015).

Case Conclusion

In this case, a 2-year-old ingested liquid nicotine that was intended for use as an electronic cigarette refill. The patient fully recovered after a period of observation without any sequelae and was discharged home the next day. As electronic cigarette use continues to grow, as will access to liquid nicotine for refilling these devices.

Specialty-Specific Guidance

Internal Medicine/Family Medicine

- Electronic cigarette refills come in various sizes and have a lot of potential for misuse, overdose, and severe toxicity in both adults and children.
- Anticipatory guidance regarding the potential dangers of these products and proper storage is important in preventing toxicity in children of parents using these products.
- Vomiting is the primary symptom seen in most patients who have ingested nicotine, but seizures can occasionally be seen as the presenting symptom in liquid nicotine ingestions.
- Children <6-year-old with possible ingestion of 1 whole cigarette or ≥3 cigarette butts should be observed in a health care setting for the development of signs of toxicity

Pediatrics

- Electronic cigarette refills come in various sizes and have a lot of potential for misuse, overdose, and severe toxicity in both adults and children.
- Anticipatory guidance regarding the potential dangers of these products and proper storage is important in preventing toxicity in children of parents using these products.
- Vomiting is the primary symptom seen in most patients who have ingested nicotine, but seizures can occasionally be seen as the presenting symptom in liquid nicotine ingestions.
- Children <6-year-old with possible ingestion of 1 whole cigarette or ≥3 cigarette butts should be observed in a health care setting for the development of signs of toxicity

Emergency Medicine

- Electronic cigarette refills come in various sizes and have a lot of potential for misuse, overdose, and severe toxicity in both adults and children.
- Vomiting is the primary symptom seen in most patients who have ingested nicotine, but seizures can occasionally be seen as the presenting symptom in liquid nicotine ingestions.
- Children <6-year-old with possible ingestion of 1 whole cigarette or ≥3 cigarette butts should be observed for development of signs of toxicity
- Patients with symptoms should be observed until asymptomatic with normal vital signs
- Clothing removal and skin decontamination should occur shortly after arrival if concerned about any dermal exposure.
- Activated charcoal is not recommended in these cases as onset of symptoms is rapid and includes vomiting and seizures in severe toxicity, making aspiration a significant risk.
- Seizures should be treated with benzodiazepines as opposed to antiepileptics. If intractable seizures, despite use of generous doses of benzodiazepines, consider barbiturates before antiepileptics.
- Treatment is primarily supportive.

Toxicology

- Electronic cigarette refills come in various sizes and have a lot of potential for misuse, overdose, and severe toxicity in both adults and children.
- Be aware of other sources of nicotine and decontamination techniques for patients exposed dermally
- Vomiting is the primary symptom seen in most patients who have ingested nicotine
- Children <6-year-old with possible ingestion of 1 whole cigarette or ≥3 cigarette butts should be observed in a health care setting for the development of signs of toxicity
- Patients with symptoms should be observed until asymptomatic with normal vital signs
- Activated charcoal is not recommended in these cases as onset of symptoms is rapid and includes vomiting and seizures in severe toxicity making aspiration a significant risk
- Seizures should be treated with benzodiazepines as opposed to antiepileptics. If intractable seizures, despite use of generous doses of benzodiazepines, consider barbiturates before antiepileptics.
- Treatment is primarily supportive.

References

Anderson MJ, Kurtycz DF, Cline JR. Baptisia poisoning: a new and toxic look-alike in the neighborhood. J Emerg Med. 2015;48(1):39–42.

Brennan R, Van Hout MC. Gamma-hydroxybutyrate (GHB): a scoping review of pharmacology, toxicology, motives for use, and user groups. J Psychoactive Drugs. 2014;46(3):243–51.

Brown MA, Guilleminault C. A review of sodium oxybate and baclofen in the treatment of sleep disorders. Curr Pharm Des. 2011;17(15):1430–5.

Caponnetto P, et al. The emerging phenomenon of electronic cigarettes. Expert Rev Respir Med. 2012;6(1):63–74.

Corkery JM, Button J, Vento AE, Schifano F. Two UK suicides using nicotine extracted from tobacco employing instructions available on the Internet. Forensic Sci Intern. 2010;199(1-3), e9–e13.

Eggleston W, Nacca N, Stork CM, Marraffa JM. Pediatric death after unintentional exposure to liquid nicotine for an electronic cigarette. Clin Toxicol (Phila). 2016;54(9):890–1.

FDA. Vaporizers, E-cigarettes, and other Electronic Nicotine Delivery Systems (ENDS). August 7, 2016. http://www.fda.gov/TobaccoProducts/Labeling/ProductsIngredientsComponents/ucm456610.htm. Accessed August 29, 2016.

Knudsen K, Greter J, Verdicchio M. High mortality rates among GHB users in western Sweden. Clin Toxicol (Phila). 2008;46(3):187–92.

Knudsen K, Jonsson U, Abrahamsson J. Twenty-three deaths with gamma-hydroxybutyrate overdose in wetern Sweeden between 2000 and 2007. Acta Anaesthesiol Scand. 2010;54(8):987–92.

Kobert R. Lehrbuch der Intoxikationen II. Band Spezieller Teil. Stuttgart: Verlag von Ferdinand Enke; 1906. p. 1064–5.

Liechti ME, Kunz I, Greminger P, Speich R, Kupferschmidt H. Clinical features of gamma-hydroxybutyrate and gamma-butyrolactone toxicity and concomitant drug and alcohol use. Drug Alcohol Depend. 2006;81(3):323–6.

Maremmani I, Lamanna F, Tagliamonte A. Long-term therapy using GHB (sodium gamma hydroxybutyrate) for treatment-resistant chronic alcoholics. J Psychoactive Drugs. 2001;33(2):135–42.

Mayer B. How much nicotine kills a human? Tracing back the generally accepted lethal dose to dubious self-experiments in the nineteenth century. Arch Toxicol. 2014;88:5–7.

Mensch AR, Holden M. Nicotine overdose after a single piece of nicotine gum. Chest. 1984;86:801–2.

Schep LJ, Slaughter RJ, Beasley DM. Nicotinic plant poisoning. Clin Toxicol (Phila). 2009;47(8):771–81.

Smolskine SC, Spoerke DG, Spiller SK, et al. Cigarette and nicotine chewing gum toxicity in children. Hum Toxicol. 1988;7:27–31.

Soghoian S. Nicotine. In: Nelson L, editor. Goldfrank's toxicologic emergencies. 9th ed. New York: McGraw-Hill; 2010. p. 1185–90.

Solarino B, Rosenbaum F, Risselmann B, Buschmann CT, Tsokos M. Death due to nicotine-containing solution: case report and review of the literature. Forensic Sci Intern. 2010;195(1-3):e19–22.

Walker N, Howe C, Glover M. Cytisine versus nicotine for smoking cessation. N Engl J Med. 2014;371(25):2353–62.

Woolf A, Burkhart K, Caraccio T, Litovitz T. Self-poisoning among adults using multiple transdermal nicotine patches. J Toxicol Clin Toxicol. 1996;34(6):691–8.

Zhu SH, Sun JY, Bonnevie E, et al. Four hundred and sixty brands of e-cigarettes and counting: implications for product regulation. Tob Control. 2014;23(Suppl 3):iii3–9.

Case 20
A Skin Rash and Fever After Starting an Antibiotic

1. Discuss common medications that are associated with Steven's Johnson Syndrome and the current understanding of their pathophysiology.
2. What is required to diagnose Steven's Johnson Syndrome?
3. What is the mechanism of methotrexate toxicity?
4. How does methotrexate toxicity commonly present? What organ systems can be involved?
5. What treatment options are available for methotrexate toxicity, and how does the renal function affect both the toxicity and the treatment strategies?
6. Does the administration of carboxypeptidase alter methotrexate concentrations?
7. What are risk factors for toxicity due to oral methotrexate?
8. What dosing errors are often cited in cases of accidental overdose?

Abstract An 87-year-old female presented to the emergency department with fever and a rash, out of concern for possible Steven's Johnson syndrome. Ultimately, it was discovered she had a medication error involving methotrexate, and the rash was felt to be due to methotrexate toxicity, rather than true Steven's Johnson syndrome. The case discusses both Steven's Johnson toxicity as well as methotrexate toxicity.

Keywords Methotrexate • Rash • Steven's Johnson • Mediation errors

L.R. Dye et al. (eds.), *Case Studies in Medical Toxicology*,
DOI 10.1007/978-3-319-56449-4_20

History of Present Illness

An 87–year-old female presented to a local emergency department for evaluation of rash and fever. The patient was in her usual state of health prior to a mechanical fall. After the fall, the patient developed rhabdomyolysis and was admitted to a rehabilitation hospital. While at the rehabilitation facility, the patient was noted to have a pruritic papular rash, gradually worsening over 1 week. Two days prior to presentation, the patient developed fever (T_{max} 39.2 C).The rehabilitation facility noted a medication error and transferred the patient to the emergency department out of concern for Stevens Johnson Syndrome. In addition to the rash, the patient complained of oral pain with resultant decreased oral intake. She denied history of similar rashes.

Past Medical History	Hypertension
	Gastroesophageal reflux disorder
	Hypothyroidism
	Paroxysmal atrial fibrillation
	Congestive heart failure
	Rheumatoid arthritis
Medications	Trimethoprim sulfamethoxazole (2 weeks prior to presentation in the emergency department)
Allergies	NKDA

Physical Examination

Blood pressure	Heart rate	Respiratory rate	Temperature	O_2 saturation
122/84 mmHg	84 bpm	18 breaths/min	36.9 °C (98.42 °F)	93%

General: Awake and alert
HEENT: White ulcers on the hard palate, excoriation of lips
Cardiovascular: Regular rate and rhythm
Pulmonary: Clear to auscultation, symmetric breath sounds
Skin: Scattered white vesicles with vesico-pustular lesions on an erythematous base
These lesions were present throughout the body, but most pronounced on the back

Diagnostic Testing

WBC	Hemoglobin	Platelets
1.1 k/mm^3 (ANC 924)	9 g/dL	57 k/mm^3

Na	K	Cl	CO_2	BUN	Cr	Glucose
136 mmol/L	3.9 mmol/L	103 mmol/L	24 mmol/L	35 mg/dL	1.1 mg/dL	152 mg/dL

AST	ALT	CK
32 IU/L	61 IU/L	28 IU/L

Lactate 0.8 mmol/L
PT 12 seconds; IR 1.1

Ancillary Testing

Chest radiograph with patchy opacities bilaterally, mild vascular congestion

Discuss Common Medications That Are Associated with Steven's Johnson Syndrome and the Current Understanding of Their Pathophysiology

Antibiotics, particularly the sulfonamides, NSAIDs, anticonvulsants such as phenytoin, and allopurinol have been associated with SJS-TEN (Stevens Johnson Syndrome-Toxic Epidermal Necrolysis) (Wetter and Camilleri 2010; French and Prins 2012). SJS & TEN are thought to occur via an immune-mediated reaction which causes widespread apoptosis of keratinocytes. This is followed by loss of viability and necrosis of the remaining epidermis (Nickoloff 2008). Antifolate cytotoxic skin reactions (i.e., methotrexate-induced toxicity) may appear similar to SJS-TEN, but are thought to occur due to direct cellular toxicity rather than an immune-mediated mechanism (Pierard-Franchimont et al. 2012).

What Is Required to Diagnose Steven's Johnson Syndrome?

The diagnosis of Steven's Johnson syndrome, like toxic epidermal necrolysis, is a clinical diagnosis, based on a combination of history and physical examination. Histologic findings on biopsy can be used to support the diagnosis, but the diagnosis is ultimately a clinical diagnosis. There is no gold-standard diagnostic laboratory test that can be ordered to confirm the diagnosis.

Hospital Course

The patient was admitted to the medical intensive care unit and treated for health care-associated pneumonia with ceftazidime and vancomycin. Leucovorin was administered for presumed methotrexate toxicity. Skin lesions were biopsied and returned negative for HSV/VZV.

On Hospital Day 2, the WBC count fell to ANC 600/mm^3 with an ANC of 348/mm^3; the platelet count fell to 8000/mm^3. The patient was transfused two single-donor apheresis platelet units. On hospital Day 4, the WBC fell to 200/mm^3. The patient was started on granulocyte colony-stimulating factor.

The patient continued to receive leucovorin, but developed worsening respiratory status with pulmonary edema and adult respiratory distress syndrome. She was started on voriconazole for possible fungal pneumonia. The patient was started on noninvasive positive pressure ventilation and diuretic therapy for fluid overload. After diuresis of 2 L, the patient developed acute kidney failure and atrial fibrillation with rapid ventricular response at 140 beats per minute.

On Hospital Day 5, the patient was intubated for worsening hypoxemic respiratory failure. Shortly thereafter, she suffered a cardiac arrest and was unable to be resuscitated.

What Is the Mechanism of Methotrexate Toxicity?

Reduced folate, i.e., tetrahydrofolate and derivatives, are required for purine and thymidine synthesis. Methotrexate enters the cell via the reduced folate carrier and ultimately undergoes polyglutamination. Methotrexate is structurally similar to folate, and methotrexate, along with the polyglutamates, inhibits dihydrofolate reductase (DHFR). This inhibition results in a depletion of reduced folates.

While synthesis of methionine and purines do not result in oxidation of tetrahydrofolate moieties, synthesis of thymidine results in oxidation to dihydrofolate, thus trapping folate in an oxidized state (Widemann and Adamson 2006; Nelson and Goldfrank 2011; Berg et al. 2002). Ultimately, there is inhibition of purine synthesis.

How Does Methotrexate Toxicity Commonly Present? What Organ Systems Can Be Involved?

Methotrexate suppresses synthesis of thymidine and purines and may result in cell death in rapidly dividing cell lines. Methotrexate toxicity may cause pancytopenia, mucositis, rash, as well as hepatitis and pneumonitis. Death may occur from pneumonia, sepsis, or multi-organ failure (Widemann and Adamson 2006; Nelson and Goldfrank 2011; Sinicina et al. 2005).

Methotrexate is primarily eliminated by the kidneys. Because methotrexate is poorly soluble at an acidic pH, methotrexate may precipitate in the renal tubules. In addition, there is some suggestion that methotrexate itself may be directly nephrotoxic to the renal tubules. This direct toxicity, along with the precipitation of methotrexate in the tubules, may result in nephrotoxicity. Renal insufficiency may increase the concentrations of methotrexate, thereby increasing the risk of systemic toxicity (Widemann and Adamson 2006).

What Treatment Options Are Available for Methotrexate Toxicity, and How Does the Renal Function Affect Both the Toxicity and the Treatment Strategies?

Supportive care, including adequate fluid resuscitation and treatment of concomitant infections, is mandatory. Urinary alkalinization may decrease the precipitation of methotrexate in the renal tubules, thereby decreasing the risk of nephrotoxicity. Folinic acid (Leucovorin) is a reduced (active) form of folic acid and can be interconverted to the various active forms of folate. Folinic acid therapy is indicated until methotrexate toxicity has resolved (Widemann and Adamson 2006; Nelson and Goldfrank 2011). Methotrexate toxicity can be considered resolved once both levels are subtherapeutic, and there is no longer any evidence of end organ toxicity.

With severe kidney dysfunction, methotrexate cannot be cleared resulting in persistently elevated concentrations, which may result in more significant toxicity. Carboxypeptidase G2 (Glucarpidase) is derived from enzymes found in Pseudomonas spp. It is recombinantly expressed in E. Coli and now is commercially available. It functions by cleaving methotrexate to DAMPA and glutamate and can rapidly lower the serum methotrexate concentration (Widemann et al. 2010).

Does the Administration of Carboxypeptidase Alter Methotrexate Concentrations?

Carboxypeptidase cleaves methotrexate into glutamate and DAMPA. DAMPA may cross react with the immunoassay for methotrexate, giving a falsely elevated concentration. The true serum methotrexate concentration can be verified by LC-MS/MS (Al-Turkmani et al. 2010).

What Are Risk Factors for Toxicity Due to Oral Methotrexate?

Interestingly, acute oral methotrexate overdose is unlikely to result in significant toxicity. This is probably because GI absorption is saturable and oral dosing is significantly lower than IV chemotherapeutic dosing (LoVecchio et al. 2008).

What Dosing Errors Are Often Cited in Cases of Accidental Overdose?

Accidental chronic overdose is a risk for significant morbidity and death. In a series reported to the FDA's AERS (Adverse Event Reporting System), the most common error leading to toxicity was confusion regarding once-weekly dosing (30% of cases) and other dosage errors (22%). Nearly one fourth of all patients in this series died. Prescribing or administration by a health care professional was responsible for 54% of errors; 19% were attributable to dispensing errors. Only 20% of errors were attributable to patient error. This series highlights the importance of due diligence in the prescribing and dispensing of methotrexate to prevent harm and potentially death (Moore et al. 2004).

Specialty-Specific Guidance

Internal Medicine/Family Medicine

- Emphasize dosing of methotrexate to patients; ensure patients know if the drug should be administered once weekly or daily
- Emphasize importance of prompt medical care should a rash occur

Dermatology

- Cytotoxic skin lesions due to methotrexate may resemble SJS-TEN, but are due to direct cellular toxicity rather than an immune-mediated phenomenon

Emergency Medicine

- Urinary alkalinization can reduce risk of toxicity
- Administer leucovorin for cases of methotrexate toxicity with normal renal function, or carboxypeptidase for cases of methotrexate toxicity with abnormal renal function

Critical Care Medicine

- Administer leucovorin for cases of methotrexate toxicity with normal renal function, or carboxypeptidase for cases of methotrexate toxicity with abnormal renal function

- Granulocyte colony-stimulating factor can be administered for drug-induced neutropenia
- A common cause of death in methotrexate toxicity is sepsis

References

Al-Turkmani MR, Law T, Narla A, Kellogg MD. Difficulty measuring methotrexate in a patient with high-dose methotrexate-induced nephrotoxicity. Clin Chem. 2010;56(12):1792–4.

Berg JM, Tymoczko JL, Stryer L. Biochemistry. 5th ed. New York: W. H. Freeman; 2002.

French LE, Prins C. Erythema multiforme, Stevens–Johnson syndrome and toxic epidermal necrolysis. 2012 [cited 3/24/2015]. In: Dermatology [Internet]. China: Elsevier Saunders; Third. [cited 3/24/2015]; p. 319–33.

LoVecchio F, Katz K, Watts D, Wood I. Four-year experience with methotrexate exposures. J Med Toxicol. 2008;4(3):149–50.

Moore TJ, Walsh CS, Cohen MR. Reported medication errors associated with methotrexate. Am J Health Syst Pharm. 2004;61(13):1380–4.

Nelson L, Goldfrank LR. Goldfrank's toxicologic emergencies. 9th ed. New York: McGraw-Hill Medical; 2011.

Nickoloff BJ. Saving the skin from drug-induced detachment. Nat Med. 2008;14(12):1311–3.

Pierard-Franchimont C, Lesuisse M, Humbert P, Delvenne P, Pierard GE. Toxic epidermal necrolysis and antifolate drugs in cancer chemotherapy. Curr Drug Saf. 2012;7(5):357–60.

Sinicina I, Mayr B, Mall G, Keil W. Deaths following methotrexate overdoses by medical staff. J Rheumatol. 2005;32(10):2009–11.

Wetter DA, Camilleri MJ. Clinical, etiologic, and histopathologic features of Stevens-Johnson syndrome during an 8-year period at Mayo Clinic. Mayo Clin Proc. 2010;85(2):131–8.

Widemann BC, Adamson PC. Understanding and managing methotrexate nephrotoxicity. Oncologist. 2006;11(6):694–703.

Widemann BC, Balis FM, Kim A, Boron M, Jayaprakash N, Shalabi A, et al. Glucarpidase, leucovorin, and thymidine for high-dose methotrexate-induced renal dysfunction: clinical and pharmacologic factors affecting outcome. J Clin Oncol. 2010;28(25):3979–86.

Case 21
Recurrent Seizures in a Patient with a Chronic Neurologic Disorder

1. Discuss the mechanism and differential diagnosis of medications that can cause multiple seizures in overdose.
2. What is 4-aminopyridine. What is it used for, and what is its mechanism?
3. What are some of the other clinical manifestations of 4-AP in overdose?
4. Discuss the role of phenytoin in the treatment of 4-aminopyridine toxicity? For what drug-induced seizures might phenytoin treatment be detrimental?
5. What are other products that contain 4-aminopyridine?
6. Why is 4 AP being investigated as a therapy in calcium channel blocker poisoning?

Abstract A 34 year-old male with an initially unknown neurologic disorder presented to the emergency department following an intentional overdose. He was initially noted to be tachycardic, somnolent, and then had a generalized tonic-clonic seizure, which appeared to have resolved, although EEG monitoring later revealed nonconvulsive status epilepticus. He was treated with multiple medications, and ultimately, made a complete recovery. A detailed discussion of drug-induced seizures, as well as the mechanism of action of this particular xenobiotic, ensues.

Keywords 4-aminopyridine • Seizures • Multiple sclerosis

L.R. Dye et al. (eds.), *Case Studies in Medical Toxicology*,
DOI 10.1007/978-3-319-56449-4_21

History of Present Illness

Chief complaint: Recurrent seizures

Emergency medical services were called to the home of a 34 year-old male with a history of a "chronic neurologic disorder" for an intentional overdose. He was in his usual state of health until the night prior, when he had an argument with his mother. He was found to be lethargic the following morning. Upon arrival of the emergency medical services, he was minimally arousable to deep stimulation, diaphoretic, and tachycardic with a maximal heart rate of 120 beats per minute. The blood pressure was 138/86 mmHg. He was transported to the emergency department.

Physical Examination

General: the patient was noted to be lethargic and somnolent. He was minimally responsive to painful stimuli.
HEENT: Pupils were 4 mm, and sluggishly reactive;
Cardiovascular: the heart rate was noted to be 120 beats per minute.
Neurologic: Spasticity of the left upper and lower extremities was appreciated and the patient was diffusely hyperreflexic.

Approximately 30 min after arrival, he was noted to have several generalized tonic-clonic seizures lasting 30–60 s, but never regained consciousness.

Initial Treatment

The patient received a total of 10 mg of intravenous lorazepam in several divided doses. He was subsequently started on a lorazepam infusion. He was intubated with succinylcholine and received 1 g of intravenous phenobarbital. The seizures terminated after he received a dose of 1 g of intravenous phenytoin. He also received 5 g of intravenous pyridoxine.

Past Medical History	"chronic neurologic disorder," but no history of seizures
Medications	Unknown at presentation
Allergies	Unknown
Family History	Unknown
Social History	Unknown

Diagnostic Testing

WBC	Hemoglobin	Platelets
17 k/mm^3	13 g/dL	300 k/mm^3

Na	K	Cl	CO_2	BUN	Cr	Glucose
143 mmol/L	3.5 mmol/L	107 mmol/L	24 mmol/L	15 mg/dL	1.2 mg/dL	169 mg/dL

AST	ALT
65 IU/L	53 IU/L

Acetaminophen, salicylates, and ethanol were undetectable
CT head: negative for hemorrhage or masses

Discuss the Mechanism and Differential Diagnosis of Medications That Can Cause Multiple Seizures in Overdose

Toxin-induced seizures can be caused either by excessive excitatory neurotransmission or lack of inhibitory signaling. Status epilepticus is defined by either two or more seizures without a lucid interval or continuous seizure activity for greater than 5 min. Toxin-induced status epilepticus is less common (Rao 2015).

Xenobiotics than can cause seizures:

• 4 aminopyridine • Antihistamines • Baclofen • Bupropion • Camphor • Carbamazepine • Carbon monoxide • Chloroquine • Cicutoxin • Cyanide • Domoic acid • Ergots • Gamma hydroxybutyrate (GHB) • Gyromitrin • Heavy metals (lead, mercury, lithium) • Hypoglycemics • Isoniazaid (INH)	• Local anesthetics • Mefanamic acid • Meperidine • Organic chlorides • Organic phosphorus compounds • Phenylbutazone • Propoxyphene • Serotonin and serotonin-norepinephrine reuptake inhibitors • Styrchnine • Sympathomimetics • Tetramethylenedisulfotetramine • Thallium • Theophylline • Tramadol • Tricyclic antidepressants • Zinc phosphide

Xenobiotics that commonly cause status epilepticus in overdose.

• 4 aminopyridine • Bupropion • Camphor • Chloroquine	• Cicutoxin • Isoniazid (INH) • Gyromitrin • Methylxanthines

Xenobiotics that commonly cause seizures in withdrawal.

• Baclofen • Barbiturates • Benzodiazepines	• Ethanol • Gamma hydroxybutyrate (GHB)

Hospital Course

The patient had a history of multiple sclerosis. His mother brought his medication list which revealed that the patient was prescribed valcyclovir, temazepam, natalizumab, and dalfampridine (4-aminopyridine or 4-AP). The patient was switched from the lorazepam drip to a propofol drip and admitted to the ICU. Continuous EEG monitoring showed intermittent nonconvulsive seizure activity until hospital day 3. The patient was extubated on hospital day 5. The 4-AP level was 530 ng/mL (therapeutic range 25–49 ng/mL). The valacyclovir level was 7.5 mcg/mL (2.0–4.0 mcg/mL). The patient was discharged on hospital day 14 with a normal mental status and neurologic exam. It was unclear if the spasticity and hyperreflexia seen in the emergency department was related to the subsequent generalized tonic-clonic seizure activity.

What Is 4-Aminopyridine. What Is It Used for, and What Is Its Mechanism?

4-aminopyridine (4-AP) is a broad-spectrum potassium channel blocker that was used in electrophysiological studies for characterizing voltage-gated potassium channels in the 1970s. These studies showed that 4-AP selectively blocked voltage-sensitive potassium channels, reduced the potassium current, and increased the action potential duration down large nerves (Blight et al. 2014). Furthermore, it was shown this only affected demyelinated nerves, with little effect on myelinated ones. In myelinated nerves, saltatory conduction down the Nodes of Ranvier leads to speedy transmission of action potentials. In MS and other demyelinating syndromes, the loss of myelin means that the strength and speed of the action potential decreases as it is propagated down long nerves. By blocking potassium efflux, the action potential can propagate more easily down demyelinated nerves. 4-AP was targeted for use in MS, as demyelination of the long nerves of the legs leads to impaired walking early in the disease course.

4-aminopyridine also increases release of acetylcholine at the neuromuscular junction, and for that reason, it has also been used in the treatment of Lambert–Eaton syndrome, myasthenia gravis, saxitoxin and tetrodotoxin-induced paralysis, anesthesia-induced neuromuscular blockade, and a botulism outbreak in Alaska with variable success (King et al. 2012).

Early studies in the 1970s through the 1990s characterized 4-AP as having a narrow therapeutic index, with an increased risk for seizures associated with higher doses (Stork and Hoffman 1994). This narrow therapeutic index represented an important barrier to clinical use. Nevertheless, 4-AP became available to some clinicians in unapproved, compounded formulations, which showed variability of dosage and resultant toxicities owing to unintended overdose (Burton et al. 2008; Schwam 2011; Stork and Hoffman 1994). However, dalfampridine (Ampyra®), a 10 mg extended release version (taken twice daily), was approved by the FDA in 2010.

Potassium channel blockade increases the resting potential of a neuron and leads to increased calcium influx and therefore increased calcium-mediated exocytosis of neurotransmitters. 4-aminopyridine is fat-soluble and can cross the blood brain barrier. It is hypothesized that in overdose, the potassium blockade affects all neurons, leading to global excitation and massive excitatory neurotransmitter release.

What Are Some of the Other Clinical Manifestations of 4-AP in Overdose?

Extrapyramidal symptoms have been described including choreoathetoid movements and slurred speech (Ballesta Méndez et al. 2014; De Cauwer et al. 2009; King et al. 2012). One case report described a 34-year-old woman with MS who developed "tremulous dystonic and choreoathetoid-type writhing of the extremities" after an intentional overdose. She was reported to have a fixed stare, slurred speech, confabulation, and delirium. She was successfully treated with lorazepam (Pickett and Enns 1996).

Various cardiac effects have been described with 4-AP toxicity and include: hypertension, supraventricular tachycardia, atrial fibrillation, bradycardia, and diffuse myocardial hypokinesis. There is a theoretical concern for QT prolongation through inhibition of the hERG potassium channel as 4-AP is a potassium channel blocker (King et al. 2012).

Discuss the Role of Phenytoin in Treatment of 4-Aminopyridine Toxicity? For What Drug-Induced Seizures Might Phenytoin Treatment Be Detrimental?

Phenytoin has been shown to help stop seizures caused by 4-aminopyridine in both case reports and animal models (Stork and Hoffman 1994; Yamaguchi and Rogawski 1992). As a sodium channel blocker, it can stop propagation of an action potential. In most toxin-induced seizures, initiation and propagation of the seizure is diffuse and does not respond to standard antiepileptic drugs such as phenytoin, and in some cases, it may theoretically be harmful. In most toxin-induced seizures, GABA-ergic agents are most effective (other than INH-induced seizures which require pyridoxine as an antidote) (Rao 2015).

What Are Other Products That Contain 4-Aminopyridine?

4-AP was initially developed in the 1960s as an avicide (Avitrol®). When consumed, 4-AP causes birds to emit distress calls secondary to involuntary diaphragmatic contractions (King et al. 2012). It is EPA-regulated as a restricted pesticide, which means it can only be used by certified commercial entities. It is highly toxic to mammals and fish. Despite restrictions on use, other animals, including household pets, have been harmed and killed by exposure to 4-AP bait each year (McLean and Khan 2013).

Why Is 4 AP Being Investigated as a Therapy in Calcium Channel Blocker Poisoning?

4-AP facilitates calcium conduction by blocking potassium channels, which causes depolarization and opening of voltage-gated calcium channels. Rodent and feline models have displayed improvement of hemodynamic outcomes with infusion doses of 2 mg/kg of 4-AP (Agoston et al. 1984; Graudins and Wong 2010; Tuncok et al. 1998). An infusion of 1 mg/kg has been effective in a dog model, but not other animal models (Gay et al. 1986). There are case reports of successful use of 4AP in CCB overdose in humans (King et al. 2012; Wilffert et al. 2007).

Specialty-Specific Guidance

Prehospital

- Bring all pill bottles to the hospital with the patient
- Provide airway support, as indicated
- Administer benzodiazepines as per local protocol

Emergency Medicine

- Early administration of benzodiazepines is indicated for seizures, with barbiturates being indicated for refractory seizures
- Unlike other toxin-induced seizures where anticonvulsants other than GABA agonists are not indicated, the administration of phenytoin or fosphenytoin may be beneficial in seizures induced by 4-AP.

- Advanced airway management, including endotracheal intubation, may be required for patients with refractory seizures

Critical Care Medicine

- Patients with 4-AP overdose may present with status epilepticus
- Phenytoin should be administered in addition to GABA agonists for 4-AP-induced seizures
- Mechanical ventilation may be required for patients with recurrent seizures following 4-AP ingestions.

References

Agoston S, Maestrone E, van Hezik EJ, et al. Effective treatment of verapamil intoxication with 4-aminopyridine in the cat. J Clin Invest. 1984;73(5):1291–6.
Ballesta Méndez M, van Pesch V, Capron A, Hantson P. Prolonged toxic encephalopathy following accidental 4-aminopyridine overdose. Case Rep Neurol Med. 2014;2014:237064.
Blight AR, Henney HR 3rd, Cohen R. Development of dalfampridine, a novel pharmacologic approach for treating walking impairment in multiple sclerosis. Ann N Y Acad Sci. 2014;1329:33–44. Review
Burton JM, Bell CM, Walker SE, O'Connor PW. 4-aminopyridine toxicity with unintentional overdose in four patients with multiple sclerosis. Neurology. 2008;71(22):1833–4.
De Cauwer H, De Wolf P, Couvreur F, et al. An unusual case of 4-aminopyridine toxicity in a multiple sclerosis patient: epileptic disorder or toxic encephalopathy? Acta Neurol Belg. 2009;109:40–1.
Gay R, Algeo S, Lee RJ, et al. Treatment of verapamil toxicity in intact dogs. J Clin Invest. 1986;77(6):1805–11.
Graudins A, Wong KK. Comparative hemodynamic effects of levosimendan alone and in conjunction with 4-aminopyridine or calcium chloride in a rodent model of severe verapamil poisoning. J Med Toxicol. 2010;6(2):85–93.
King AM, Menke NB, Katz KD, Pizon AF. 4-aminopyridine toxicity: a case report and review of the literature. J Med Toxicol. 2012;8(3):314–21.
McLean MK, Khan S. A review of 29 incidents involving 4-aminopyridine in non-target species reported to the ASPCA animal poison control center. J Med Toxicol. 2013;9(4):418–21.
Pickett TA, Enns R. Atypical presentation of 4-aminopyridine overdose. Ann Emerg Med. 1996;3:382–5.
Rao R. Chapter 24: Neurologic principles. In: Hoffman RS, et al., editors. Goldfrank's toxicologic emergencies. 10th ed. New York: McGraw Hill Education; 2015.
Schwam E. Severe accidental overdose of 4-aminopyridine due to a compounding pharmacy error. J Emerg Med. 2011;41(1):51–4.
Stork CM, Hoffman RS. Characterization of 4-aminopyridine in overdose. J Toxicol Clin Toxicol. 1994;32(5):583–7.
Tuncok Y, Apaydin S, Gelal A, et al. The effects of 4-aminopyridine and bay K 8644 on verapamil-induced cardiovascular toxicity in anesthetized rats. J Toxicol Clin Toxicol. 1998;36(4):301–7.
Wilffert B, Boskma RJ, van der Voort PH, et al. 4- Aminopyridine (fampridine) effectively treats amlodipine poisoning: a case report. J Clin Pharm Ther. 2007;32(6):655–7.
Yamaguchi S, Rogawski MA. Effects of anticonvulsant drugs on 4-aminopyridine-induced seizures in mice. Epilepsy Res. 1992;11(1):9–16.

Case 22
Caustic Ingestion in a Toddler

1. What kind of agent is responsible for her injury?
2. What is the mechanism of injury after caustic ingestion?
3. What is used to clean deep fryers/frying pans?
4. What are the consequences of a caustic ingestion? What organ systems are affected?
5. How should the clinician approach the patient with caustic ingestion?

Abstract A 3–year-old girl ingests a cleaning product in her home which is intended for use in the industrial setting. The clinical effects, workup, and management of caustic ingestions are discussed.

Keywords Caustic toxicity • Sodium hydroxide • Pediatrics ingestion

History of Present Illness

A 3-year-old girl spies some white powder on her mother's frying pan in the kitchen. Thinking it is sugar, she runs her forefinger through the powder and licks her finger. She immediately starts to feel discomfort and starts crying. The regional Poison Control Center is contacted, where the staff has just seen a media report of the same substance causing severe illness in an adult accidentally ingesting the product. The child is referred directly to the closest ED.

L.R. Dye et al. (eds.), *Case Studies in Medical Toxicology*,
DOI 10.1007/978-3-319-56449-4_22

On further history, her father works at a nearby restaurant and uses this cleaning product obtained through a restaurant supplier. He brought it home to use because it is more effective than household cleaners to de-grease frying pans and deep fryers.

Past Medical History	None
Medications	None
Allergies	None
Family History	Non-contributory
Social History	Lives with her parents and infant sibling

Physical Examination

Blood pressure	Heart rate	Respiratory rate	Temperature	O_2 saturation
100\55 mmHg	99 bpm	20 breaths/min	37.4 °C (99.3 °F)	90% (4 L)

General: awake, crying but consolable
HEENT: swelling of both lips with erythema (Fig. 1); linear burn in middle of tongue, consistent with contact made by licking finger
Cardiovascular: normal
Pulmonary: no rhonchi or wheezing, normal work of breathing
Abdomen: soft, non-tender, non-distended
Skin: no other signs of burns

Ancillary Testing

Chest x-ray demonstrates no evidence of pneumomediastinum.
Soft tissue neck x-ray demonstrates no airway edema.

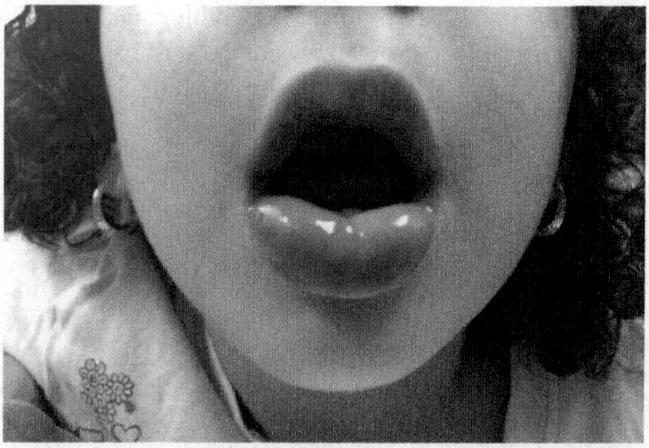

Fig. 1 External examination revealing focal swelling and mild erythema of lips

Hospital Course

She was admitted to the pediatrics floor and made NPO; endoscopy was performed the following day demonstrating no injury distal to the tongue, including the hypopharynx and esophagus.

Key Points of Case

What Kind of Agent is Responsible for Her Injury?

Cleaning product ingestion is among the most common poison exposures reported in children annually (Mowry et al. 2014), owing in large part to the availability within the home. Young children, primarily between 1 and 5 years of age, are often curious without caution—they do not yet have the reasoning skills to prevent them from ingesting a potentially dangerous household toxin. This is made especially worse when the substance is removed from its original container, or as in this case, when the substance is not intended for household use at all but is packaged at an industrial strength.

The majority of cleaning products causing toxic injury in children are caustics, usually strong acids or alkalis. Other toxic chemicals in the home include hydrocarbons (e.g., gasoline, torch oil, potpourri oil), toxic alcohols (such as antifreeze or windshield washer fluid), and pesticides. Table 1 provides a list of commonly available household toxins.

The potential for severe injury from a caustic product is most determined by the product's pH, concentration, and the amount ingested. The formulation also plays a role, as a thin liquid may be more likely to cause damage throughout the esophagus and stomach, whereas a highly viscous solid may only cause oral injury. A powder such as this one can either cause local injury alone or, if sufficient quantity is ingested, can cause distal injury as well.

What Is the Mechanism of Injury After Caustic Ingestion?

Tissue injury from a caustic ingestion begins immediately, thus limiting the benefit of any decontamination measures. Although histologic patterns of injury are different based on whether the product is acid or alkali, the clinical consequences are similar. Nonetheless, alkalis cause a liquefactive necrosis and theoretically induce deeper tissue injury (Arévalo-Silva et al. 2006). Acids, on the other hand, cause coagulation necrosis which some authors suggest limit further tissue penetration and injury via eschar formation (Browne and Thompson 2003). Unlike alkali ingestions, acids may be associated with a higher incidence of systemic complications including renal failure, liver dysfunction, disseminated intravascular coagulation, and hemolysis.

Table 1 Common toxic household chemicals

Caustics	
Acids	Toilet bowl cleaner—sulfuric or phosphoric acid Oven cleaner—sulfuric acid Tile cleaners—muriatic (hydrochloric) acid Brake dust cleaner—hydrofluoric acid
Alkali	Drain cleaner— Sodium or potassium hydroxide Bleach Ammonia Fryer cleaner—sodium hydroxide
Concentrated detergents	Laundry detergent pods Laundry detergent powder
Hydrocarbons	
Petroleum distillates	Gasoline, kerosene, lighter fluid, naphtha
Other essential oils	Pine oil, citronella oil (tiki torch fluid), potpourri oil, teak oil
Aromatic hydrocarbons	Inhalants—screen cleaners, correction fluid, paint thinner
Toxic alcohols	
Ethylene glycol	Automotive antifreeze
Methanol	Windshield washer fluid, Sterno fuel
Pesticides	
Rodenticides	Long-acting anticoagulant, "superwarfarins"
Organophosphates, carbamates	Insecticides
Pyrethroids	Insecticides

What Is Used to Clean Deep Fryers/Frying Pans?

There are a number of industrial cleaning products available to clean deep fryers, usually available in a white powdered form. The week before this case presented to our medical center, a woman sustained severe caustic injury at a restaurant when, by report, the iced tea provided was accidentally mixed with fryer cleaner instead of sugar (McFall 2014). In that case, the product was a highly concentrated sodium hydroxide (>60%) formulation.

The parents of this child provided the name of this product (Clean Force Fryer Cleaner™), and review of the Material Safety Data Sheet (MSDS) shows the powder to contain 67% Sodium Hydroxide (Fig. 2). The concentration clearly identifies it as an industrial use product.

In contrast, household cleaners containing sodium hydroxide, often referred to as "lye," are required to be in much more dilute form. For example, household drain cleaners, which can still cause significant caustic injury if ingested, contain approximately 2–4% sodium hydroxide.

```
1.2  Product Type: Powdered High Alkaline Cleaner
1.3  Hazard Rating:  Health:   3     Fire:   0     Reactivity:   1
---------------------------------------------------------------------------
       Substances Subject to SARA 313 Reporting Are Indicated by "#"
---------------------------------------------------------------------------
```

2.0 HAZARDOUS COMPONENTS / (in mg/m3)

		CAS No.	%	PEL	TWA
2.1	Sodium hydroxide (caustic soda)	1310-73-2	67	2	2C
2.2	Potassium hydroxide (caustic potash)	1310-58-3	4	No	2C
2.3	Sodium carbonate (soda ash)	497-19-8	5-20	No	No
2.4	Sodium linear alkyl benzene sulfonate	25155-30-0	3	No	No

```
---------------------------------------------------------------------------
STEL = ACGIH short term exp. limit (15 min)      PEL = OSHA 8 hr ave in air
TWA = ACGIH 8 hr average              C = ceiling limit in air, do not exceed
---------------------------------------------------------------------------
```

3.0 PHYSICAL DATA /

Fig. 2 Material Safety Data Sheet (MSDS) for product ingested

What Are the Consequences of a Caustic Ingestion? What Organ Systems Are Affected?

After ingestion of a caustic substance, immediate injury occurs to the tissues with which it comes into contact. This can include the face, lips, tongue, oropharynx, larynx, esophagus, and stomach. Ocular exposure should also be considered. Patients can have burns and swelling at all of these sites, the most immediately life-threatening being the airway.

Other consequences which occur in the first hours to day after exposure can include esophageal burns, perforation, mediastinitis, and gastric burns and perforation.

Patients may develop shock and systemic inflammation due to tissue injury or occult perforation. Acid ingestions in particular may cause a metabolic acidosis due to absorption of the offending substance into the circulation.

Subsequently, in the days to weeks following exposure, the patient is at risk for late-onset perforation, esophageal stricture, and long-term risk of esophageal carcinoma.

How Should the Clinician Approach the Patient with Caustic Ingestion?

The initial focus should be as always on basics of life support—establishing the patency of the airway and absence of airway injury, determining the patient's respiratory status and evaluating for the presence of shock.

The patient should be assessed for stridor as well as signs of aerodigestive tract injury. Patients may have drooling, vomiting, hematemesis, and respiratory distress. Chest and neck radiographs should be obtained to determine the presence of pneumomediastinum and laryngeal injury, respectively, in patients with fever, respiratory distress, or an otherwise severe clinical presentation.

Endoscopy is essential in any patient in whom there has been a significant ingestion, or in whom there are any symptoms of caustic tissue injury. Even patients with only one or two symptoms, such as drooling and refusal to eat, are at risk of esophageal injury (Crain et al. 1984). Exceptions to this rule may include patients who ingest dilute household bleach or ammonia, or products whose high viscosity prevents them from causing distal injury (crème hair relaxers). Laundry detergent pod exposures are a unique circumstance in which the need for endoscopy is controversial, as discussed in Chapter 1.

Any patient whose workup reveals suspected viscus perforation should have an immediate surgical evaluation. Caustic mediastinitis and/or peritonitis are grave diagnoses which demand immediate intervention. Empiric antibiotics are only indicated in the case of suspected perforation, but are often administered due to the patient's ill appearance and the presence of fever. Corticosteroids may prevent stricture formation in patients with moderate esophageal burns without overt necrosis (Usta et al. 2014; Anderson et al. 1990). Although benefit has not been shown in historical studies (Anderson), a recent study demonstrated a reduction in stricture formation in children with second-degree esophageal burns (Usta et al. 2014).

Case Conclusion

Following endoscopy, the patient was given a clear diet and advanced to solids over the next 24 h. She tolerated this and was discharged home the following day.

Specialty-Specific Guidance

Pediatrics

- Even small caustic exposures can result in significant injury
- Of the many cleaning substances available in the home, be aware of those with caustic ingredients such as drain and porcelain cleaners.
- Other potential household chemicals with toxic properties include hydrocarbons, pesticides, and alcohols.
- After caustic ingestion, immediate referral to the emergency department is essential for assessment of the airway and staging of esophageal injury.

Emergency Medicine

- Although caustic ingestions primarily cause esophageal and gastric injury, initial assessment must evaluate the airway for injury.
- Obtain a chest radiograph to exclude mediasitinitis or overt perforation.

- Beware of ingestions of industrial strength caustics which have a much higher likelihood to cause severe esophageal and gastric injury.

Gastroenterology

- Early flexible endoscopy is essential to determine the extent of esophageal and gastric injury in any symptomatic patient who has ingested a caustic product.
- Patients with moderate esophageal burns may benefit from corticosteroids, according to recent evidence.

Toxicology

- Fryer cleaners are most often concentrated bases, such as sodium hydroxide. This is especially the case with industrial products.
- Any patient with either a suicidal ingestion or symptoms of esophageal or laryngeal injury, even if mild, should undergo flexible endoscopy.
- Following endoscopy, corticosteroids appear to have a role in moderate esophageal injury.
- While antibiotic therapy is less established based on the available literature, it is often employed due to the patients' ill appearance and concern for micro- or overt perforation.

References

Anderson KD, Rouse TM, Randolph JG. A controlled trial of corticosteroids in children with corrosive injury of the esophagus. N Engl J Med. 1990;323:637–40.

Arévalo-Silva C, Eliashar R, et al. Ingestion of caustic substances: a 15-year experience. Laryngoscope. 2006;116:1422–6.

Browne J, Thompson J. Caustic ingestion. In: Bluestone CD, Stool SE, Kenna MA, editors. Pediatric otolaryngology. 4th ed. Philadelphia: WB Saunders; 2003. p. 4330–42.

Crain EF, Gershel JC, Mezey AP. Caustic ingestions. Symptoms as predictors of esophageal injury. Am J Dis Child. 1984;138:863–5.

McFall, M. Poisoned tea traced to sugar mixup; Utah victim critical. The Salt Lake Tribune. 2014. www.sltrib.com.

Mowry JB, Spyker DA, Cantilena LR, et al. 2013 Annual report of the American association of poison control centers' National Poison Data System (NPDS): 31st Annual report. Clin Toxicol. 2014;52:1032–283.

Usta M, Erkan T, Cokugras FC, et al. High doses of methylprednisolone in the management of caustic esophageal burns. Pediatrics. 2014;133:E1518–24.

Case 23
Withdrawal from Chronic Headache Medication

1. What is the differential diagnosis?
2. What is the mechanism of action of cyproheptadine and how is it used therapeutically?
3. What are side effects of cyproheptadine use?
4. How common is cyproheptadine withdrawal syndrome?
5. What is serotonin syndrome?
6. Which patients are at risk of developing serotonin syndrome?
7. How does cyproheptadine play a role in the management of serotonin syndrome?
8. What are symptoms of barbiturate withdrawal?
9. What are symptoms of baclofen withdrawal?
10. What are symptoms of opioid withdrawal?
11. What are some general management principles for patients with symptoms of withdrawal?

Abstract This chapter delves into the case of an 8-year-old male who develops withdrawal symptoms after a chronic headache medication is discontinued. Multiple withdrawal syndromes are reviewed, as well as general management principles of withdrawal.

Keywords Cyproheptadine • Baclofen withdrawal • Barbiturate withdrawal • Serotonin syndrome

L.R. Dye et al. (eds.), *Case Studies in Medical Toxicology*,
DOI 10.1007/978-3-319-56449-4_23

History of Present Illness

An 8-year-old male presented to the emergency department via EMS for evaluation of agitation, which developed after waking in the morning. The mother reported the patient had become increasingly agitated and sweaty after waking to the point she was unable to calm him, so she called EMS. The patient had been healthy and without complaints the previous day. The only change reported by his mom was that he received the last dose of his daily, chronic headache medication 36 h prior to his current symptoms. He had been on this medication for the past 2.5 months. The mother called the pharmacy for a medication refill when the bottle was empty, but had not realized she was running low on the medication prior to that point, and the pharmacy was out of stock of the medication. The pharmacist noted it would be several days before the medication would be available. As the patient's mother did not like the sedating effect of the medication, she decided to discontinue it altogether.

The patient had not been sick prior to the onset of symptoms and denied headache.

Past Medical History	Chronic headaches
Medications	Daily headache medication—mother unable to recall name
Allergies	NKDA
Social History	Lives at home with parents and siblings No history of behavioral issues Some new stressors were noted at home.
Family History	Unknown, patient was adopted.

Physical Examination

Blood pressure	Heart rate	Respiratory rate	Temperature	O_2 saturation
146/84 mmHg	110 bpm	21 breaths/min	37 °C (98.6 °F)	97% (room air)

General: Awake, agitated.
Cardiovascular: Tachycardic, no murmurs, gallops or rubs.
Respiratory: Tachypnea, no stridor or audible wheezing.
Abdomen: Soft, no apparent tenderness, non-distended. Active bowel sounds appreciated.
Neurological: Awake, alert, agitated. No focal deficits. No clonus, no hyperreflexia, normal muscular tone.
Skin: Mildly and diffusely diaphoretic.

Diagnostic Testing

Na	K	Cl	CO_2	BUN/Cr	Glucose
139 mmol/L	3.6 mmol/L	106 mmol/L	25 mmol/L	16/0.51 mg/dL	95 mg/dL

Comprehensive drug screen (serum) via GC/MS: caffeine and theobromine—positive; ibuprofen 31 mcg/mL

Ancillary Testing

EKG: normal sinus rhythm, rate 96 bpm, PR 115 ms, QRS 78 ms, QTc 434 ms

What Is the Differential Diagnosis?

- Discontinuation syndrome
- Clonidine withdrawal
- Opioid withdrawal
- Baclofen withdrawal
- Barbiturate withdrawal from chronic use of medication containing acetylsalicylic acid/butalbital/caffeine
- Behavioral issues
- Intoxication by medications or substances belonging to others in the home

Hospital Course

In the emergency department, he was quickly calmed with verbal direction and was given 1 mg of lorazepam orally. His symptoms improved, and after a brief observation period, and he was discharged home.

Second ED Visit

Later that evening, approximately 48 h after the last dose of his headache medication, he became increasingly agitated, inconsolable, and began throwing things. EMS was called again. Due to his significant agitation, he received midazolam 2 mg IV from EMS and lorazepam 2 mg IV on arrival to the emergency department.

Physical Examination

Blood pressure	Heart rate	Respiratory rate	Temperature	O_2 saturation
115/69 mmHg	120 bpm	20 breaths/min	37.2 °C (98.9 °F)	99% (room air)

General: Patient was screaming and not directable,
Cardiac: Tachycardic, limited exam due to agitation
Pulmonary: No stridor, wheezing, rales or accessory muscle use
Abdominal: Soft, ND, NT. Bowel sounds present
Neurologic: Awake, agitated and not directable. Normal reflexes, no rigidity, and no clonus
Skin: Mildly diaphoretic

On this presentation, the patient's mother was uncertain of the dosing for the medication, but wrote down the name of the medication prior to calling EMS. She reported the patient was taking cyproheptadine for his headaches. She was uncertain of the dose, but thought it was 4 mg twice a day.

Hospital Course

The poison center was called and recommended giving the patient his home dose of cyproheptadine. Within 30 min of receiving the medication, the patient became calm and went to sleep. He was observed overnight and discharged in the morning with plans to resume cyproheptadine 4 mg twice daily.

Third ED Visit

Within a few hours of discharge, the patient had another escalation in his behavior (72 h after last dose of his prescribed cyproheptadine). He was again out of control, unable to sit still, and sweating. He returned to ED by EMS. The patient required 5-point restraints and was given olanzapine 5 mg IM.

At this point, the patient's home dosing regimen was by the patient's pharmacy. He had been taking cyproheptadine 8 mg twice daily, not 4 mg twice daily as mom had originally thought. He received 8 mg cyproheptadine orally in the ED, and within 30 min, he had fallen asleep. He was admitted to the hospital and had no recurrence of his symptoms. He was discharged safely from the ED with a plan for a prolonged taper of cyproheptadine.

What Is the Mechanism of Action of Cyproheptadine and How Is It Used Therapeutically?

- Cyproheptadine is a first-generation antihistamine. It is an H1 blocker that also exhibits nonspecific 5HT antagonism.
- Currently, cyproheptadine is most commonly used to treat serotonin toxicity (Lappin and Auchincloss 1994; Graudins et al. 1998).
- Cyproheptadine is also used as an appetite stimulant for children with poor growth and cystic fibrosis patients, as well as children with functional gastrointestinal disorders (Homnick et al. 2004; Madani et al. 2015; Mahachoklertwattana et al. 2009). Additional uses include male and female anorgasmia with TCA therapy, and for prophylaxis of child/adolescent migraines (Decastro 1985; Lewis 2004; McCormick et al. 1990; Eiland et al. 2007; Bille et al. 1977).
- Dosing guidelines for cyproheptadine vary depending on the use. Some authors describe a daily maximum dose of up to 32 mg/day. For serotonin receptor antagonism, Kapur et al. report 95% blockade of 5-HT2 receptors in the pre-frontal cortex on PET scanning with dosing of 18 mg/day (6 mg three times daily) (Kapur et al. 1997). Previous manuscripts documenting use of cyproheptadine to treat migraines used dosing of 0.2–0.4 mg/kg/day for pediatric patients and 2 mg twice daily for patients 17–53 years of age (Bille et al. 1977; Rao et al. 2000).

What Are Side Effects of Cyproheptadine Use?

- Cyproheptadine is an older medication used rarely in daily practice, in part due to its side effect profile.
- Reported side effects with routine use include sedation, increased appetite, and central anticholinergic syndrome (Blaustein et al. 1995; Watemberg et al. 1999).
- Case reports of cyproheptadine overdose include descriptions of classic anticholinergic toxicity (tachycardia, psychomotor agitation, delirium) (Baehr et al. 1986; Richmond and Seger 1985).

How Common Is Cyproheptadine Withdrawal Syndrome?

- There are only two other cases reported in the literature (De Lucas Taracena et al. 2000; Bhatia et al. 2015).
- The case presented by De Lucas et al. is not referred to in most pediatric textbooks or articles reviewing cyproheptadine and associated side effects.

What Is Serotonin Syndrome?

- Serotonin syndrome is a constellation of symptoms caused by serotonin excess. It is characterized by:
  - The presence of at least one serotonergic agent;
  - Autonomic instability (for example, hyperthermia, GI distress, diaphoresis, or tachycardia);
  - CNS involvement (for example, clonus, altered mental status, or psychomotor agitation).
- There are several decision rules that can be used to define serotonin syndrome. Sternbach's Criteria has been used historically, but many toxicologists currently refer to The Hunter Criteria (Sternbach 1991; Dunkley et al. 2003).
- Serotonin syndrome is a potentially life-threatening diagnosis and should be recognized quickly.

What are the Hunter Criteria?

To meet the Hunter Criteria for serotonin syndrome, patients must have exposure to a serotonergic agent and one of the following (Dunkley et al. 2003):

- Spontaneous clonus
- Inducible clonus AND agitation or diaphoresis
- Ocular clonus AND agitation or diaphoresis
- Tremor AND hyperreflexia
- Hypertonia AND temperature >38C AND ocular clonus OR inducible clonus

Which Patients Are at Risk of Developing Serotonin Syndrome?

- Serotonin syndrome most frequently occurs when patients take multiple medications with activity at the serotonin receptor.
- Specifically, patients are affected when additional serotonergic medications are added to a medication regimen with existing serotonergic medications or when the dosage of a long-term medication is increased.
- Serotonin syndrome is also reported in cases of accidental and intentional overdose of multiple drugs with serotonergic properties.

How Does Cyproheptadine Play a Role in the Management of Serotonin Syndrome?

- Cyproheptadine has been used in the treatment of serotonin syndrome because of its 5HT (serotonin) receptor antagonism.
- It is believed cyproheptadine counteracts the effects of serotonin excess by blocking the serotonin receptor.
- While the literature describes some success controlling symptoms of serotonin syndrome, cyproheptadine is an adjunctive therapy to other supportive measures such as benzodiazepines, cooling, and hydration.

What Are Symptoms of Barbiturate Withdrawal?

- Agitation, hallucinations, and altered mental status
- Hypertension
- Tachycardia
- Diaphoresis
- Hyperthermia
- Seizures

What Are Symptoms of Baclofen Withdrawal?

- Altered mental status, hallucinations
- Hypertension
- Tachycardia
- Tremor
- Seizures
- Occasionally, can see hypotension and bradycardia

What Are Symptoms of Opioid Withdrawal?

- Nausea, vomiting, diarrhea
- Piloerection
- Diaphoresis
- Abdominal pain/cramping

What Are some General Management Principles for Patients with Symptoms of Withdrawal?

- Management of withdrawal symptoms is based on the specific drug involved.
- Abrupt discontinuation of baclofen, benzodiazepine, or barbiturates can lead to medically significant withdrawal symptoms, seizures, and death. A tapered discontinuation of the drug is recommended.
- Selective serotonin reuptake inhibitor discontinuation can lead to a syndrome that is typically not life-threatening, but can be unpleasant. A tapered discontinuation is also recommended.
- Opioid withdrawal is typically not life-threatening, but is very uncomfortable for patients. Medications like alpha-2 antagonists, anti-diarrheal agents, and anti-emetics are often used to assist with symptoms of withdrawal.
- Longer acting medications such as methadone and buprenorphine are sometimes used to treat patients with opioid dependence. Not only do these medications help control withdrawal symptoms, but they help combat cravings due to their activity at the mu receptor.

Case Conclusion

In this case, the patient was experiencing withdrawal effects from the discontinuation of cyproheptadine. Previously, this medication was used for the treatment of chronic headaches in the pediatric patient, but is rarely used for this indication today. For this patient, his symptoms improved when the medication was restarted and a gradual taper initiated.

Specialty-Specific Guidance

Internal Medicine/Family Medicine

- Consider side effects when starting patients on long-term medications
- Familiarize yourself with risks of withdrawal syndromes from any prescribed medications and advise patients accordingly when discontinuing a medication.
- Some medications that have known withdrawal syndromes are baclofen, barbiturates, benzodiazepines, opioids, and selective serotonin reuptake inhibitors.
- If you have questions about the potential for a medication to cause withdrawal symptoms, call your local poison control center or discuss the medication with your local toxicologist.

Pediatrics

- Consider side effects when starting patients on long-term medications
- Familiarize yourself with risks of withdrawal syndromes from any prescribed medications and advise patients accordingly when discontinuing a medication.
- Some medications that have known withdrawal syndromes are baclofen, barbiturates, benzodiazepines, opioids, and selective serotonin reuptake inhibitors.
- If you have questions about the potential for a medication to cause withdrawal symptoms, call your local poison control center or discuss the medication with your local toxicologist.

Emergency Medicine

- Reviewing all home medications, supplements, and vitamins that patients have access to is extremely important when evaluating overdose and patients with withdrawal syndromes.
- Always consider discontinuation of medication as a possible cause of symptoms.
- Just as intoxication is considered as a potential cause of agitation or delirium, withdrawal syndromes should also be considered when evaluating the agitated or delirious patient.
- Some medications that have known withdrawal syndromes are baclofen, barbiturates, benzodiazepines, opioids, and selective serotonin reuptake inhibitors.
- Patients with active sings of withdrawal from benzodiazepines, baclofen, and barbiturates often require admission.
- In many cases, restarting the offending agent and providing a taper for discontinuation is the best choice.
- If the potential for a medication to cause withdrawal symptoms is in question, call the local poison control center or discuss the medication with your local toxicologist.

Toxicology

- The differential diagnosis for altered mental status should include withdrawal or discontinuation syndromes
- Consider unusual or infrequently seen medications when assessing patients with signs of drug toxicity or histories suggestive of a withdrawal syndrome.
- In many cases, restarting the offending agent and providing a taper for discontinuation is the best choice.
- Contacting a patient's pharmacy can be very helpful when trying to determine home medications

References

Baehr GR, Romano M, Young JM. An unusual case of cyproheptadine (Periactin) overdose in an adolescent female. Pediatr Emerg Care. 1986;2(3):183–5.

Bhatia MS, Kaur J, Gautam P. A case of serotonin syndrome following cyproheptadine withdrawal. Prim Care Companion CNS Disord. 2015;17(3). doi:10.4088/PCC.14l01762.

Bille B, Ludvigsson J, Sanner G. Prophylaxis of migraine in children. Headache. 1977;17:61–3.

Blaustein BS, Gaeta TJ, Balentine JR, Gindi M. Cyproheptadine-induced central anticholinergic syndrome in a child: a case report. Pediatr Emerg Care. 1995;11(4):235–7.

Decastro R. Reversal of MAOI-induced anorgasmia with cyproheptadine. Am J Psychiatry. 1985;142(6):783.

De Lucas Taracena MT, Alcaina Prosper T, Huélamo Ortega MJ. Psychotic syndrome after withdrawal of cyproheptadine: remission with olanzapine. Actas Esp Psiquiatr. 2000;28(4):270–2.

Dunkley EJ, Isbister GK, Sibbritt D, Dawson AH, Whyte I. The hunter serotonin toxicity criteria: simple and accurate diagnostic decision rules for serotonin toxicity. QJM. 2003;96(9):635–42.

Eiland LS, Jenkins LS, Durham SH. Pediatric migraine: pharmacologic agents for prophylaxis. Ann Pharmacother. 2007;41(7):1181–90.

Graudins A, Stearman A, Chan B. Treatment of the serotonin syndrome with cyproheptadine. J Emerg Med. 1998;16(4):615–9.

Homnick D, Homnick B, Reeves A, et al. Cyproheptadine is an effective appetite stimulant in cystic fibrosis. Pediatr Pulmonol. 2004;38(2):129–34.

Kapur S, Zipursky R, Jones C, et al. Cyproheptadine: a potent in vivo serotonin antagonist. Am J Psychiatry. 1997;153(6):884.

Lappin R, Auchincloss E. Treatment of the serotonin syndrome with cyproheptadine. N Engl J Med. 1994;331:1021–2.

Lewis DW, Diamond S, Scott D, Jones V. Prophylactic treatment of pediatric migraine. Headache. 2004;44(3):230–7.

Madani S, Cortes O, Thomas R. Cyproheptadine use in children with functional gastrointestinal disorders. J Pediatr Gastroenterol Nutr. 2015. [Epub ahead of print].

Mahachoklertwattana P, Wanasuwankul S, Poomthavorn P, Choubtum L, Sriphrapradang A. Short-term cyproheptadine therapy in underweight children: effects on growth and serum insulin-like growth factor-I. J Pediatr Endocrinol Metab. 2009;22(5):425–32.

McCormick S, Olon J, Brotman A. Reversal of fluoxetine induced anorgasmia by cyproheptadine in two patients. J Clin Psychiatry. 1990;51:383–4.

Rao B, Das D, Taraknath V, Sarma Y. A double blind controlled study of propranolol and cyproheptadine in migraine prophylaxis. Neurol India. 2000;48:223–6.

Richmond M, Seger D. Central anticholinergic syndrome in a child: a case report. J Emerg Med. 1985;3(6):453–6.

Sternbach H. The serotonin syndrome. Am J Psychiatry. 1991;148:705–13.

Watemberg NM, Roth KS, Alehan FK, Epstein CE. Central anticholinergic syndrome on therapeutic doses of cyproheptadine. Pediatrics. 1999;103(1):158–60.

Case 24
Weakness in a Dialysis Patient

1. What are the signs and symptoms of digoxin toxicity?
2. What is the mechanism of digoxin toxicity?
3. What medications were prescribed that may enable digoxin toxicity?
4. What treatment should be pursued at this time?
5. How does digoxin Immune Fab work?
6. How is digoxin immune Fab dosing calculated in chronic toxicity?
7. Does renal dysfunction change management?
8. What special monitoring should take place once a patient has received digoxin immune Fab?
9. Are there alternatives to aid in the clearance of digoxin that does not involve renal metabolism in the anuric patient?
10. Is there a preferred timing for administration of digoxin immune Fab and undergoing plasmapheresis?
11. Are there cost advantages to the use of plasmapheresis versus repeated administration of digoxin immune Fab?

Abstract Digoxin toxicity usually arises due to increased dosing, impaired clearance, or interaction with other concomitant medications. Cardiac dysrhythmias may result, and the most effective treatment is the administration of digoxin-specific antibody. However, once the antibody is administered, renal clearance is required to eliminate the drug-antibody complex from the circulation. In patients with anuric renal failure, additional treatment modalities such as plasmapheresis may be needed to avoid recurrent toxicity once the antibody dissociates from the drug.

Keywords Digoxin • Plasmapheresis for toxicology • Immunoglobulin Fab fragments

L.R. Dye et al. (eds.), *Case Studies in Medical Toxicology*,
DOI 10.1007/978-3-319-56449-4_24

Case

A 78-year-old dialysis-dependent man with digoxin toxicity.

History of Present Illness

A 78-year-old man with a complex medical history on hemodialysis presents to the Emergency Department after 2 days of worsening weakness, nausea, and visual abnormalities. He reports difficulty walking from the parking lot to the store over the last 2 days, and that this morning's generalized weakness was severe enough that he could not sit up in bed. He has felt nauseated the entire time; however, there has been no emesis. In regard to his vision, he reports that staring at lights results in bright, fuzzy spots.

The patient was recently discharged from the hospital on levofloxacin and vancomycin following a bout of hospital-associated pneumonia as well as surgical graft infection. He has atrial fibrillation and takes digoxin 0.125 mg three times a week after hemodialysis.

Past Medical History	End-stage renal disease on dialysis, congestive heart failure, heart block status post-pacer placement, coronary artery disease, diabetes mellitus, cerebrovascular accident, deep venous thrombosis, and gastrointestinal bleeding
Medications	Lantus, digoxin, midodrine, lispro, amiodarone, levothyroxine, simvastatin, tamusolin
Allergies	Cefazolin, hydrocodone, neomycin
Family History	Father with heart attack and mother with stroke history
Social History	Former smoker, denies recreational drug use or alcohol consumption

Physical Examination

Blood pressure	Heart rate	Respiratory rate	Temperature	O_2 saturation
97/47 mmHg	74 bpm	16 breaths/min	36.5 °C (97.7 °F)	100% (room air)

General: No acute distress. Alert, pleasant, interactive, and communicative. Mild cachexia

Head: Mild temporal wasting.

Eyes: Pupils equal, round, and constricted.

ENT: moist mucous membranes.

Neck: Supple, no JVD.

Cardiovascular: Regular rate and rhythm. 3/6 harsh systolic blowing murmur.

Pulmonary: Clear to auscultation bilaterally. Normal effort.

Abdomen: Soft, distended with chronic epigastric tenderness, no rebound.
Extremities: 1+ pitting edema to knees bilaterally.
Neurologic: Awake, alert, and oriented to person, place, time. Mild dysarthria.

Diagnostic Testing

Sodium 131 mEq/L, Potassium 4.9 mEq/L, Creatinine 5.56 mg/dL
Digoxin 12 ng/mL.

Ancillary Testing

EKG: Wide complex, Paced rhythm.

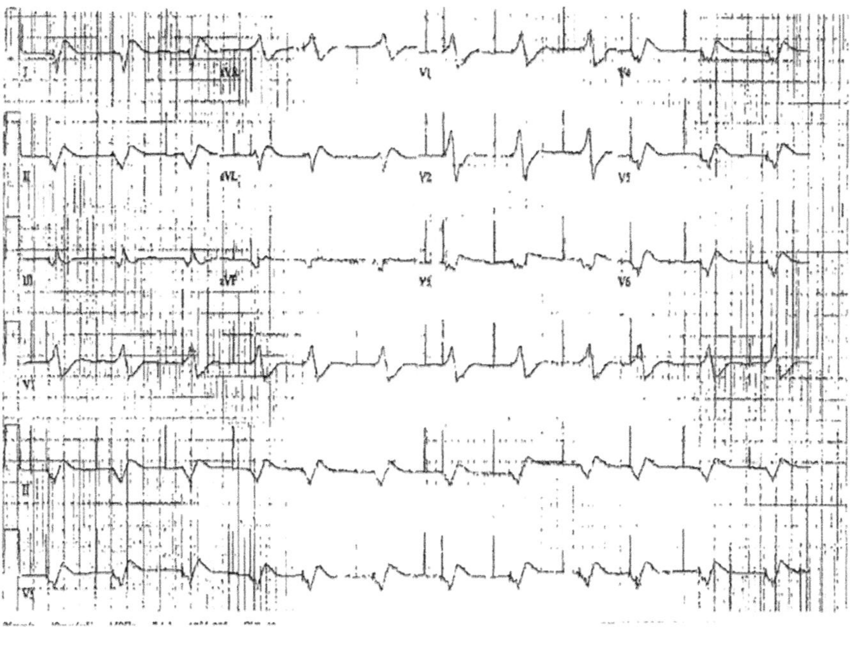

What Are the Signs and Symptoms of Digoxin Toxicity?

Digoxin toxicity is typically described in terms of cardiac and extra-cardiac symptoms. Extra-cardiac symptoms include visual disturbances (i.e., haziness or blurring of vision, flashing lights, halos and/or color disturbances), fatigue, anorexia, nausea, vomiting and hallucinations (Bauman et al. 2006; Critchley and Critchley 1997). Regarding cardiac manifestations, sinus bradycardia is the most common, but malignant dysrhythmias are the most concerning manifestation. Digoxin toxicity reportedly causes nearly every rhythm disturbance. That said, dysrhythmias that should alert the clinician to digoxin toxicity include: new-onset Mobitz type I AV block, accelerated junctional rhythm with or without high-degree AV block, non-paroxysmal atrial tachycardia with AV block, and bidirectional ventricular tachycardia. Dysrhythmias not attributable to digoxin toxicity may include any supraventricular tachycardia with a rapid ventricular response and Mobitz type II AV block (Bauman et al. 2006).

What Is the Mechanism of Digoxin Toxicity?

Digoxin's therapeutic effect is derived from increasing intracellular calcium in the cardiac myocyte. This is accomplished by inhibition of the transmembrane Na-K ATPase pump, which in turn eliminates the sodium gradient needed for calcium efflux at the Na-Ca antiporter. This results in an increase in cytosolic calcium, the substrate for the cell's contractile apparatus. In therapeutic dosing, digoxin increases myocardial contractility and stroke volume. The drug also has chronotropic and dromotropic effect as increased intracellular calcium raises the resting membrane potential, slowing conduction through the SA and AV nodes, but enhancing automaticity and shortening repolarization intervals. For this reason, the drug is used both to increase contractility in heart failure and to prevent rapid conduction of supraventricular dysrhythmias.

In excess dosing, the chronotropic and dromotropic effects are exaggerated. Sinus bradycardia or atrioventricular block is common, and the myocardium becomes irritable and prone to dysrhythmias. On the ECG, this may manifest as QTc interval shortening and scooped ST segments, often referred to as the "digitalis effect."

What Medications Were Prescribed that May Enable Digoxin Toxicity?

Digoxin is a substrate for p-glycoprotein, a membrane-bound transporter present in many organ systems including the gastrointestinal (GI) tract, central nervous system, and kidneys. In the GI tract, p-glycoprotein is capable of effluxing drug molecules, thereby limiting drug absorption and systemic circulation. In the kidney, p-glycoprotein increases the excretion of drug molecules into the urine. As a result, chemicals that inhibit p-glycoprotein function may increase the serum concentration levels of digoxin. For example, co-administration of digoxin with known p-glycoprotein inhibitors (e.g., amiodarone, verapamil, and quinidine) may increase serum digoxin concentrations by enhancing intestinal absorption and decreasing renal clearance (Bauman et al. 2006). This patient is on amiodarone, which may have increased his risk for digoxin toxicity.

What Treatment Should Be Pursued at This Time?

In the setting of severe digoxin toxicity, the administration of digoxin immune Fab (DIGIBIND®, DigiFab™) may be lifesaving. In the current case, the patient presenting with hyperkalemia at a level of 4.9 mEq/L and a digoxin level of 12.0 ng/mL suggests significant symptoms of severe toxicity. The presence of cardiac dysrhythmias is likely masked by the patient's pacemaker and should not preclude administration of the antidote.

How Does Digoxin Immune Fab Work?

Digoxin immune Fab is a specific antidote for digoxin. It is extracted from the serum of sheep that have been immunized with a digoxin-hapten complex. The Fab fragment is separated via enzymatic degradation to yield smaller, less antigenic and more mobile molecules that are able to bind digoxin and quickly remove digoxin from its active binding site; thus isolating it within the extracellular compartment (Ujhelyi et al. 1993).

How Is Digoxin Immune Fab Dosing Calculated in Chronic Toxicity?

The number of immune Fab vials (40 mg apiece) to fully reverse digoxin toxicity can be calculated using the following formula:

$$\text{Dose}\left(\#\ \text{of vials}\right) = \frac{\text{Digoxin concentration}\left(\text{ng}/\text{mL}\right) \times \text{Patient's weight}\ \left(\text{kg}\right)}{100}$$

In an unstable patient in which the digoxin concentration is not yet known, an empiric administration of 6 vials is an alternative regimen.

Patients utilizing digoxin therapy are likely suffering from significant underlying disease. Sudden complete reversal may lead to acute decompensation of their previously controlled symptoms. Partial reversal, reduction in the total dose by 20–25%, has been advocated as a way to treat the toxicity, while continuing to control the patient's underlying disease.

For this patient:

$$\text{Calculated Dose}\left(\#\ \text{of vials}\right) = \frac{12\ \text{ng}/\text{mL} \times 65\ \text{kg}}{100} = 7.8\,\text{vials}$$

The calculated dose for complete reversal would have been 8 vials; however, given the concern for decompensation of his known atrial fibrillation as well as congestive heart failure, a partial reversal (i.e., reduction by 25%) of 5–6 vials was ultimately recommended.

Does Renal Dysfunction Change Management?

Renal metabolism is primarily responsible for the clearance of digoxin as well as the digoxin/digoxin immune Fab complex. Thus, renal dysfunction leads to impaired clearance of both digoxin and the digoxin/digoxin immune Fab complex (Ujhelyi et al. 1993). Studies evaluating whether age and renal impairment alter digoxin pharmacokinetics suggest that there should be no dosing changes in the elderly and/or renal impaired (Renard et al. 1997). In the setting of end-stage renal disease, renal failure results in no clearance of the digoxin/digoxin immune Fab, and a rebound of the free digoxin occurs in 1–8 days. This rebound results in return of symptoms and may require re-dosing of digoxin immune Fab. (Ujhelyi et al. 1993, Rabetoy et al. 1990)

What Special Monitoring should Take Place Once a Patient Has Received Digoxin Immune Fab?

The digoxin/digoxin Fab complex is not pharmacologically active, and thus, measurements of the complex do not provide insight into active digoxin levels. The classical measurement of a digoxin concentration tends to elevate significantly after digoxin Fab administration since it is measuring the free digoxin in addition to the digoxin/digoxin immune Fab complex. Therefore, accurate measurements should look at free digoxin concentration; however, this testing is not commonly performed, and the clinician needs to contact laboratory personnel to ensure that it is available and results returned in a clinically relevant time frame (Ujhelyi et al. 1993).

Case Continued

In the management of this particular patient, the poison center recommended monitoring free digoxin levels to better assess his pharmacologic burden. One day after admission and administration of six vials of digoxin immune Fab, the patient's digoxin levels increased to 32.9 ng/mL; however, free digoxin level were only 1.1 ng/mL. At this time, the patient had complete resolution of symptoms, as demonstrated by resolution of nausea, improvement in abdominal pain, and ability to read as well as walk independently to the bathroom. Review of his pill counts as well as his medication history revealed that the patient had mistakenly taken his digoxin three times daily for several days, rather than three times weekly.

Are There Alternatives to Aid in the Clearance of Digoxin That Does Not Involve Renal Metabolism in the Anuric Patient?

Some cases have evaluated the use of plasmapheresis or plasma exchange for the management of digoxin toxicity. Plasmapheresis involves the removal of the digoxin/digoxin immune Fab complex from the plasma where it has been sequestered in those unable to really excrete the complex (Rabetoy et al. 1990; Zdunek et al. 2000).

Another method for management of digoxin toxicity in the setting of renal failure involves charcoal intestinal dialysis, or multi-dose activated charcoal. In charcoal intestinal dialysis, a high intraluminal concentration of charcoal creates a gradient between the plasma and the intestinal lumen, allowing the redistribution and binding of the drug into the charcoal. Additional data suggest that digoxin may undergo active secretion into the intestines; thus, charcoal may prevent further reabsorption (Critchley and Critchley 1997).

Case Continued

At this time, the poison center recommended considering multi-dose activated charcoal and plasmapheresis with his next hemodialysis to aid in the removal of digoxin/digoxin immune Fab complex. On the fourth day of admission, the patient's symptoms returned in spite of having received one round of plasmapheresis with his last hemodialysis. At this time, repeated laboratory studies revealed a free digoxin level 2.2 ng/mL, which increased to 2.7 ng/mL upon repeat evaluation. Quantification of total digoxin level was found to be 22.6 ng/mL, and upon repeat testing, it was down to 12.5 ng/mL; thus demonstrating a dissociation effect of the digoxin/digoxin immune Fab complexes in this anuric patient.

Is There a Preferred Timing for Administration of Digoxin Immune Fab and Undergoing Plasmapheresis?

Although data is limited, it is theorized that the timing of plasmapheresis to digoxin immune Fab dosing should reflect the time to peak of bound digoxin levels. Thus, plasmapheresis would be best performed within 1–3 h of administration of digoxin immune Fab so as to trap as much of the complex in the plasma just prior to removal (Zdunek et al. 2000).

Are There Cost Advantages to the Use of Plasmapheresis Versus Repeated Administration of Digoxin Immune Fab?

The cost of digoxin immune Fab varies by institution; however, it is reported to be in the range of $2725 per 40 mg vial (Lexicomp 2015). The cost of plasmapheresis again varies by institution, but published reports suggest a cost of $4099. This cost includes both a round of plasmapheresis and the replacement albumin required as part of the treatment (Heatwole et al. 2011). Thus, if a patient requires re-dosing, with a minimum of two vials of digoxin immune Fab, the cost of the antidote would already outweigh the cost of one round of plasmapheresis. Digoxin toxicity is rarely encountered in the setting of hemodialysis-dependent end-stage renal disease; however, the use of plasmapheresis ideally within 3 h of digoxin immune Fab administration may provide a cost advantage compared to repeated dosing of immune Fab.

Case Conclusion

Recommendations by the poison center included repeated dosing of digoxin immune Fab with three more vials, as well as a plasmapheresis session within 3 h of digoxin immune Fab administration. After re-dosing of digoxin immune fab and subsequent plasmapheresis, the patient's symptoms resolved, and his free digoxin levels were found to be 1.8 ng/mL. The patient was observed overnight with no symptoms and was discharged without digoxin as a prescription.

Specialty-Specific Guidance

Toxicology

- Ensure that anuric patients treated with digoxin immune Fab are monitored for signs and symptoms of complex dissociation in the next 1–8 days.
- Patients need re-dosing of digoxin immune Fab if symptoms return.
- Monitor free digoxin concentrations.
- Consider alternative clearance modalities in anuric patients
  - Plasmapheresis
  - Multi-dose-activated charcoal

Nephrology

- Evaluate the appropriateness of digoxin therapy in hemodialysis patients given difficult clearance.
- Consider medical toxicologist consultation in setting of elevated digoxin levels.
- Consider the use of plasmapheresis in the setting of elevated digoxin levels when patient undergoes their next hemodialysis session.

References

Bauman JL, Didomenico RJ, Galanter WL. Mechanisms, manifestations, and management of digoxin toxicity in the modern era. Am J Cardiovasc Drugs. 2006;6(2):77–86.

Critchley JA, Critchley LA. Digoxin toxicity in chronic renal failure; treatment by multiple dose activated charcoal intestinal dialysis. Hum Exp Toxicol. 1997;16:733–5.

Heatwole C, Johnson N, Holloway R, Noyes K. Plasma exchange vs. intravenous immunoglobulin for myasthenia gravis crisis: an acute hospital cost comparison study. J Clin Neuromuscul Dis. 2011;13(2):85–94.

Lexicomp. Digoxin Immune Fab. Pricing: US. 2015 Accessed 02 Sept 2015.

Rabetoy GM, et al. Treatment of digoxin intoxication in a renal failure patient with digoxin-specific antibody fragments and plasmapheresis. Am J Nephrol. 1990;10:518–21.

Renard C, Grene-Lerouge N, Beau N, Baud F, Scherrmann JM. Pharmacokinetics of digoxin-specific Fab: effects of decreased renal function and age. Br J Clin Pharmacol. 1997;44(2):135–8.

Ujhelyi MR, Robert S, Cummings DM, Colucci RD, Green PJ, Sailstad J, et al. Influence of digoxin immune Fab therapy and renal dysfunction on the disposition of total and free digoxin. Ann Intern Med. 1993;119:273–7.

Zdunek M, Mitra A, Mokrzycki MH. Plasma exchange for the removal of digoxin-specific antibody fragments in renal failure: timing is important for maximizing clearance. Am J Kidney Dis. 2000;36(1):177–83.

Case 25
Hyperlactemia

1. What is the differential diagnosis for hyperlactemia?
2. Why was the patient's lactate elevated?
3. What clinical findings suggest clenbuterol toxicity?
4. What is propofol infusion syndrome?
5. Describe key features of cyanide toxicity.
6. How does cyanide cause lactate elevation?
7. What are other mitochondrial toxins that should be considered and how do they cause lactic acidosis?
8. How do antifreeze products cause an increase in lactate levels?
9. Should lactic acidosis be treated with parenteral bicarbonate?
10. What are some non-toxicologic causes of elevated lactate concentrations?

Abstract In this case, an 18-year-old male presents to the emergency department with status asthmaticus. He subsequently developed hyperlactemia during the first 8 h of his hospitalization. This chapter reviews causes of hyperlactemia, including specific discussions on propofol infusion syndrome, toxic alcohol-related hyperlactemia, clenbuterol exposure, and mitochondrial toxins.

Keywords Hyperlactemia • Theophylline • Albuterol • Cyanide toxicity

L.R. Dye et al. (eds.), *Case Studies in Medical Toxicology*,
DOI 10.1007/978-3-319-56449-4_25

History of Present Illness

An 18-year-old male presented to the emergency department by EMS with a severe asthma exacerbation. He reported the acute onset of shortness of breath while playing basketball. He denied recent illness, fever, rhinorrhea, sore throat, or chills. He denied recreational drug use or known exposure to chemicals/fumes.

Past Medical History	Asthma
Medications	Albuterol inhaler Montelukast
Allergies	NKDA
Social History	Denies tobacco, ethanol, or other drugs of abuse College student who works as a sales clerk in a clothing store

Physical Examination

Blood pressure	Heart rate	Respiratory rate	O_2 saturation
163/80 mmHg	135 bpm	27 breaths/min	81% on NRB 15 L

General: He was in extremis with significant respiratory distress.
Skin: Warm, mildly diaphoretic, slightly mottled.
Pulmonary: Wheezing appreciated in all lung fields with visible accessory muscle use and tachypnea. No stridor.
Cardiovascular: Tachycardic; No murmurs, gallops, or rubs.
Abdomen: Soft, non-tender, non-distended with normal active bowel sounds.
Extremities: Atraumatic, no edema.
Neurologic: Awake, alert, anxious but oriented to person and place. No gross focal deficits.

Hospital Course

In attempts to avoid intubation, the patient was administered continuous albuterol nebulization, subcutaneous epinephrine, methylprednisolone, magnesium sulfate, and intravenous theophylline. Ultimately, he was intubated for respiratory failure, but continued to have poor aeration and wheezing throughout all lung fields. While intubated and paralyzed, the patient continued to receive intravenous theophylline and aerosolized albuterol every 30 min. He was sedated with fentanyl and midazolam infusions.

The critical care team was initially concerned about possible cyanide poisoning as further laboratory studies showed venous hyperoxia, and the patient had an increasing lactic acid concentration over an 8-h period. Toxicology was consulted and evaluated the patient 10 h after intubation.

Physical Exam at Time of Toxicology Consultation

Blood pressure	Heart rate	Respiratory rate	O_2 saturation
122/50 mmHg	118 bpm	18 breaths/min	100% on vent

General: Intubated, paralyzed, and sedated.
Skin: Warm and dry. Normal color.
Cardiovascular: Tachycardia with no murmurs, gallops, or rubs noted. 2+ pulses appreciated in all four extremities.
Pulmonary: Diffuse wheezing throughout all lung fields, but air movement was appreciated throughout.
Abdominal: Abdomen soft, non-tender and non-distended. Normal active bowel sounds.
Neurologic: GCS 3 T.

Diagnostic Testing

Na	K	Cl	CO_2	BUN/Cr	Glucose
140 mEq/L	3.2 mEq/L	102 mEq/L	21 mEq/L	11/0.9 mg/dL	172 mg/dL

Theophylline level: 7.5 μg/mL
ABG: pH 7.18, pCO2 57, pO2 121, oxygen saturation 99%
Venous oxygen saturation: 98%
Lactate: 7.6 mmol/L

What Is the Differential Diagnosis for Hyperlactemia?

- Tissue or gut ischemia
- Propofol infusion syndrome
- Metformin toxicity
- Massive ibuprofen overdose

- Propylene glycol toxicity
- Methanol ingestion
- Clenbuterol toxicity
- Beta agonism effect (with a left to right shunt)
- Phosphine gas exposure
- Direct mitochondrial toxin
  - Cyanide toxicity
  - Sodium azide toxicity
  - Hydrogen sulfide toxicity
  - Dinitrophenol exposure

Hospital Course Continued

Over the next 6 h, the patient's respiratory status improved, and nebulized albuterol treatments and theophylline administration were tapered off. As the adrenergic medications were weaned, the patient's lactate concentration improved. Twelve hours following the discontinuation of theophylline and albuterol, his lactate was 0.2 mmol/L, and his pH 7.4 with a pCO2 43 and pO2 46 on venous blood gas.

Why Was the Patient's Lactate Elevated?

- Prior to intubation, the patient received a number of adrenergic medications that likely contributed to the development of his hyperlactatemia.
- Patients receiving high doses of β-agonist can have significantly elevated lactate levels (Dodda and Spiro 2012; Manthous 2001; Maury et al. 1997; Stratakos et al. 2002).
- Hyperlactemia from β-agonists has been reported in the literature and has been reproduced in human studies (Rodrigo and Rodrigo 2005; Phillips et al. 1980).
- This phenomenon tends to occur within the first several hours of treatment.
- A prospective study of patients presenting to an ED with acute severe asthma exacerbations found elevated serum albuterol level to be a predictor of elevate lactate level. Hyperlactemia did not correlate with either increased rate of hospitalization or lower FEV1 at 3 h for patients in this study (Lewis et al. 2014).
- There are cases reported in the literature where this elevation in lactate may have led to an interim worsening of the patient's clinical course as patients compensated for the lactate-associated metabolic acidosis (Dodda and Spiro 2012; Prakash and Mehta 2002)
- Decreasing and ultimately discontinuing β-agonist therapy leads to reduction of and resolution of hyperlactemia.

- The exact physiology has not been identified, but primarily suspected to be directly related to a β-mediated effect on cellular metabolism (Chasiotis et al. 1983)
- Specifically, increased glycogenolysis and glycolysis, which releases lactate from skeletal muscle, may be the cause of β-agonist-induced elevation in plasma lactate concentrations (Chasiotis et al. 1983).

What Clinical Findings Suggest Clenbuterol Toxicity?

- Clenbuterol is a β3-agonist used by body builders, illegally as a weight loss supplement, and illegally to bulk up cattle (Daubert et al. 2007; Ramos et al. 2004)
- It has also been found as an adulterant in illicit drugs such as heroin (Hoffman et al. 2001; Hoffman et al. 2008)
- Symptoms of toxicity include:
  - Tachycardia
  - Nausea and diarrhea
  - Tremors
  - Hypertension
  - Leukocytosis
  - Hypokalemia

What Is Propofol Infusion Syndrome?

- A syndrome that develops in patients on prolonged infusions of propofol (Bray 1998; Kang 2002).
- Patients develop notable metabolic acidosis with lactate elevation, which is thought to be caused by altered metabolism/utilization of free fatty acids by mitochondria.
- Patients can have cardiac dysrhythmias and often develop a right bundle branch block
- Other symptoms include:
  - Muscle deterioration with evidence of myoglobinuria or rhabdomyolysis
  - Bradycardia resistant to treatment that can progress to asystole
  - Lipemia

Describe Key Features of Cyanide Toxicity.

- Typically, there is a very rapid onset (seconds to minutes) of clinical effects from the time of cyanide exposure.
- However, the time to development of toxicity from compounds that are metabolized to cyanide, such as amygdalin or linamarin (cyanogenic glycosides), is slower.

- There is no classic toxidrome, but neurologic and cardiovascular symptoms are most prominent with cyanide toxicity. These include:
  - Altered mental status such as agitation and confusion
  - Seizures
  - Coma
  - Hypotension and bradycardia
- GI symptoms such as abdominal pain, nausea, and vomiting can occur with ingestions of cyanide salts in addition to the neurologic and cardiovascular symptoms.
- Laboratory findings include:
  - Significantly elevated lactate (>10 mmol/L)
  - Metabolic acidosis with an anion gap
  - Venous hyperoxia

How Does Cyanide Cause Lactate Elevation?

- Movement of hydrogen ions across the inner mitochondrial membrane via cytochrome a3 of the electron transport chain is one of the vital last steps in producing ATP.
- Cyanide inhibits the activity of cytochrome oxidase at cytochrome a3 in the electron transport chain, which ultimately inhibits ATP production.
- If ATP cannot be produced, anaerobic respiration ensues and lactate is generated from pyruvate resulting in hyperlactemia.

What Are Other Mitochondrial Toxins That Should Be Considered and How Do They Cause Lactic Acidosis?

- There are a number of mitochondrial toxins other than cyanide.
- Carbon monoxide, methanol, phosphine gas, and sodium azide are all mitochondrial toxins and specifically inhibit cytochrome aa3.
- Salicylates, dinitrophenol, and pentachlorophenol are mitochondrial toxins that are electron transport chain uncouplers.
- Rotenone, a plant-derived fish poison, is an NADH-CoQ reductase inhibitor. When NADH-CoQ reductase is inhibited, so is electron transport chain activity.
- Any interference inhibition of electron transport chain activity inhibits oxidate metabolism.
- By inhibiting oxidative metabolism, cells are forced to rely on anaerobic metabolism, where the conversion of pyruvate to lactate generates a small amount of ATP.
- An increase in circulating lactate is one of the most notable effects of mitochondrial toxins.

How Do Antifreeze Products Cause an Increase in Lactate Levels?

- Ethylene glycol
  - Ethylene glycol is metabolized to glycolate and oxalate.
  - In severe cases, patients poisoned with EG can have a high lactate concentration.
  - This detection in elevated lactate is a false positive. Some laboratory assays actually detect glycolate as lactate.
  - The cross reactivity in the assay is due to the similarity in structure between glycolate and lactate.
  - There is a linear relationship between glycolate concentration and the false positive lactate concentration (Manini et al. 2009).
- Propylene glycol
  - Propylene glycol is sold as environmental-friendly antifreeze.
  - It is also used as a diluent for many intravenous medications (examples: etomidate, lorazepam, phenytoin, diazepam).
  - Propylene glycol is metabolized to lactic acid. Normally, the liver converts lactate to pyruvate via the Cori cycle.
  - In large ingestions of propylene glycol, lactate concentrations may be high and may remain high due to decreased ability to convert lactate to pyruvate.
  - This same effect is noted in critically ill patients receiving a significant amount of medication containing propylene glycol as the diluent. One example would be a patient receiving high doses of lorazepam for sedation during mechanical ventilation.
  - If patients have normal hepatic and renal function, they can quickly clear the lactate once the offending agent is discontinued. For patients with renal and hepatic failure, clearance is prolonged, and in rare cases, hemodialysis to assist in lactate removal may be recommended.

Should Lactic Acidosis Be Treated with Parenteral Bicarbonate?

- There is no definitively correct answer for this question.
- Studies do not show any benefit in increasing responsiveness to catecholamines in patients treated with sodium bicarbonate for academia (Forsythe and Schmidt 2000).
- Using parenteral bicarbonate to treat lactic acidosis can cause (Forsythe and Schmidt 2000):
  - Increased intracranial pressure
  - Fluid overload
  - Electrolyte abnormalities

- Hyperosmolality
- Worse outcomes in patients with septic shock (Boyd and Walley 2008)
- Some providers, however, feel there may be benefits of treating lactic acidosis with sodium bicarbonate, even if it is a temporizing measure and not definitive treatment. (Forsythe and Schmidt 2000; Kraut and Kurtz 2001)

What Are Some Non-toxicologic Causes of Elevated Lactate Concentrations?

- Seizure
- Shock with poor perfusion
- Ischemia (mesenteric or limb)
- Liver dysfunction
- Inborn errors of metabolism
- Thiamine deficiency
- Ketoacidosis

Case Conclusion

In this case, the patient presented with status asthmaticus. He was treated aggressively with β-agonists while in the emergency department and subsequently intubated for respiratory failure. During the first several hours of his hospitalization, he continued to receive multiple β-agonists and developed hyperlactemia. In this case, the lactate elevation was related to the β-agonists and not another exposure. The patient's hyperlactemia resolved with the discontinuation of β-agonist therapy and he fully recovered.

Specialty-Specific Guidance

Internal Medicine/Family Medicine

- Continue to prescribe β-agonists to your patients, but be clear regarding dose and frequency administration.
- Patients requiring home albuterol treatments more frequently than prescribed should be evaluated by a physician or other healthcare provider.
- Hospitalized patients receiving large amounts of β-agonists such as albuterol or theophylline may develop lactic acidosis.

- In general, as a patient's β-agonist requirement decreases, his/her lactic acidosis should resolve. Patients with renal failure do not clear lactate as readily and may have delayed improvement in lactic acidosis.
- There are many potential causes for hyperlactemia which should be reviewed with every case of significantly elevated lactate to ensure no missed diagnoses.

Pediatrics

- Continue to prescribe β-agonists to your patients, but be clear regarding dose and frequency of administration.
- Patients requiring home albuterol treatments more frequently than prescribed should be evaluated by a physician or other healthcare provider.
- Hospitalized patients receiving large amounts of β-agonists such as albuterol or theophylline may develop lactic acidosis.
- In general, as a patient's β-agonist requirement decreases, his/her lactic acidosis should resolve. Patients with renal failure do not clear lactate as readily and may have delayed improvement in lactic acidosis.
- There are many potential causes for hyperlactemia which should be reviewed with every case of significantly elevated lactate to ensure no missed diagnoses.
-

Emergency Medicine

- A detailed history of illness and medication history needs to be taken.
- In addition, be cognizant of those patients requiring a significant amount of β-agonists when in extremis, as they may develop a lactic acidemia.
- The treatment for lactic acidemia in the setting of β-agonist use is supportive.
- There is little role for parenteral sodium bicarbonate therapy.
- As the patient's β-agonist requirement decreases, their lactic acid concentrations should also decrease.
- Recognize that some parenteral pharmaceuticals can cause lactic acidosis in addition to other agents.

Toxicology

- It is important to always obtain a thorough history of present illness, home medication history, social history (specifically hobbies of all those living in the home), and details of any possible environmental exposures.

- Always review all medications administered to the patient while in the hospital.
- If a patient is found to have a profound lactic acidemia, other etiologies such as clenbuterol toxicity, propofol infusion syndrome, excessive propylene glycol use, or cyanide toxicity should be considered.

References

Boyd JH, Walley KR. Is there a role for sodium bicarbonate in treating lactic acidosis from shock? Curr Opin Crit Care. 2008;14:379–83.

Bray RJ. Propofol infusion syndrome in children. Paediatr Anesthe. 1998;8:491–9.

Chasiotis D, Sahlin K, Hultman E. Regulation of glycogenolysis in human muscle in response to epinephrine infusion. J Appl Physiol Respir Environ Exerc Physiol. 1983;54(1):45–50.

Daubert GP, Mabasa VH, Leung VW, et al. Acute clenbuterol overdose resulting in supraventricular tachycardia and atrial fibrillation. J Med Toxicol. 2007;3:56–60.

Dodda V, Spiro P. Can albuterol be blamed for lactic acidosis? Respir Care. 2012;57(12):2115–8.

Forsythe SM, Schmidt GA. Sodium bicarbonate for the treatment of lactic acidosis. Chest. 2000;117(1):260–7.

Hoffman RJ, Hoffman RS, Freyberg CL, et al. Clenbuterol ingestion causing prolonged tachycardia, hypokalemia, and hypophosphatemia with confirmation by quantitative levels. J Toxicol Clin Toxicol. 2001;39:3390–44.

Hoffman RS, Kirrane BM, Marcus SM, Clenbuterol Study Investigators. A descriptive study of an outbreak of clenbuterol-containing heroin. Ann Emerg Med. 2008;52(5):548–53.

Kang TM. Propofol infusion syndrome in the critically ill patient. Ann Parmacother. 2002;36:1453–6.

Kraut A, Kurtz I. Use of base in the treatment of severe acidemic states. Am J Kidney Dis. 2001;38(4):703–27.

Lewis LM, Ferguson I, House SL, et al. Albuterol administration is commonly associated with increases in serum lactate in patients with asthma treated for acute exacerbation of asthma. Chest. 2014;145(1):53–9.

Manini AF, Hoffman RS, McMartin KE, Nelson LS. Relationship between serum glycolate and falsely elevated lactate in severe ethylene glycol poisoning. J Anal Toxicol. 2009;33(3):174–6.

Manthous C. Lactic acidosis in status asthmaticus. Chest. 2001;119:1599–602.

Maury E, Ioos V, Lepecq B, et al. A paradoxical effect of bronchodilators. Chest. 1997;111(6):1766–7.

Phillips PJ, Vedig AE, Jones PL, et al. Metabolic and cardiovascular side effects of the β2-adrenoceptor agonists salbutamol and rimiterol. Br J Clin Pharmacol. 1980;9:483–91.

Prakash S, Mehta S. Lactic acidosis in asthma: report of two cases and review of the literature. Can Respir J. 2002;9(3):203–8.

Ramos F, Silveira I, Silva JM, et al. Proposed guidelines for clenbuterol food poisoning. Am J Med. 2004;117:362.

Rodrigo GJ, Rodrigo C. Elevated plasma lactate level associated with high dose inhaled albuterol therapy in acute severe asthma. Emerg Med J. 2005;22:404–8.

Stratakos G, Kalomenidis J, Routsi C, Papiris S, Roussos C. Transient lactic acidosis as a side effect of inhaled salbutamol. Chest. 2002;122(1):385–6.

Case 26
Tachycardia in a Patient from an Opioid Detoxification Facility

1. What medications can induce torsades and what medications can be used to treat torsades?
2. Describe the substance suspected and its history.
3. What is the rationale for using this substance for opioid detoxification?
4. What is the typical dose of this substance and the typical detoxification regimen?
5. Is this substance legal in the United States?
6. What is the proposed mechanism of action?
7. What are potential toxicities associated with this substance?

Abstract The patient is a 63-year-old male who presented from an opioid detoxification facility after he was found to be tachycardic. He was started on a relatively unique opiate detoxification regimen, which included ibogaine. On physical exam in the emergency department, however, he was bradycardic, but otherwise asymptomatic. Shortly after arrival, he developed torsade de pointes. This case discusses drug-induced torsades, as well as detailed discussion of ibogaine.

Keywords Ibogaine • Opioid detoxification • Bradycardia • Torsades

History of Present Illness

63-year-old male presents to the emergency department from an opioid detoxification facility after he was noted to be tachycardic with a maximal heart rate of 200 beats per minute, prompting emergency medical services to be called. He was previously healthy without any significant past medical history, except for opioid abuse

L.R. Dye et al. (eds.), *Case Studies in Medical Toxicology*,
DOI 10.1007/978-3-319-56449-4_26

at the time he entered the detoxification facility. Prior to entering the detoxification facility, he had been on a methadone maintenance program, where he was receiving 34 mg of methadone daily. However, he had stopped this 1 month prior to his presentation to his current presentation. Three days prior to his emergency department presentation, he was started on an immediate release morphine regimen of 50 mg daily, and 15 h prior to the current presentation, he was started on a pharmacologic detoxification regimen.

Past Medical History	Opioid abuse
Medications	Denies
Allergies	No known drug allergies
Social History	Past history of opioid abuse. + tobacco.

Physical Examination

Blood pressure	Heart rate	Respiratory rate	Temperature	O_2 saturation
110/70 mmHg	40 bpm	16 breaths/min	37 °C (98.6 °F)	99% (room air)

General: Awake and alert
Cardiovascular: Bradycardic rhythm
Pulmonary: Clear breath sounds
Abdomen: Soft and non-tender
Pulses: Palpable dorsalis pedis and radial pulses that were equal and symmetric
Neurologic: Normal

Emergency Department Course

Upon arrival in the emergency department, he was noted to be bradycardic with a heart rate of 36. He had QT prolongation, with a corrected QT interval of 498 ms (Fig. 1). Shortly thereafter, he had two episodes of torsade de pointes, associated with loss of consciousness (Fig. 2). In addition, he had multiple additional episodes of pause-dependent ventricular tachycardia. At least one of these episodes was associated with myoclonic jerking versus possible seizure activity. The patient was given 2 g of intravenous magnesium and was admitted to the critical care unit.

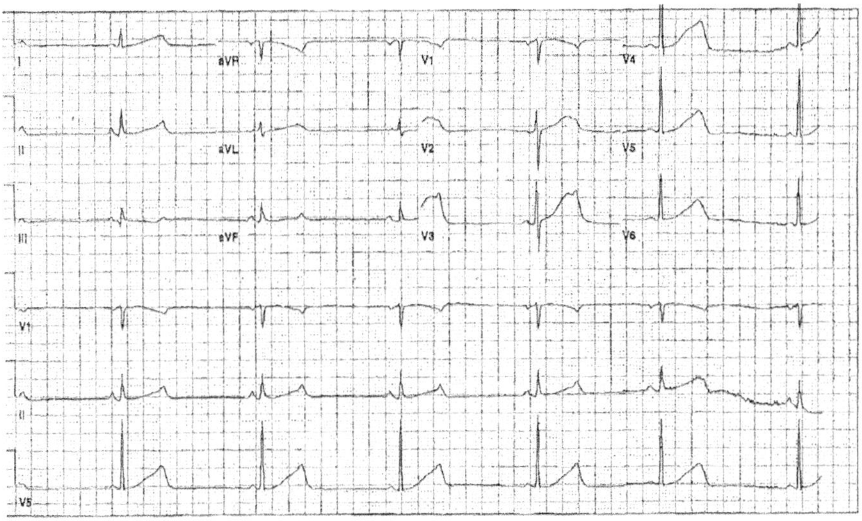

Fig. 1 Initial emergency department EKG

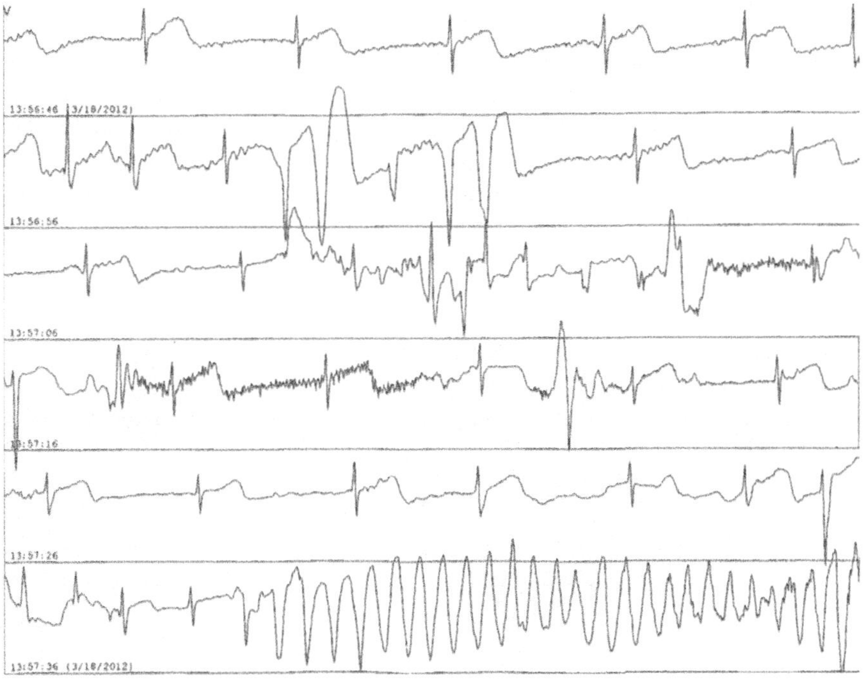

Fig. 2 Telemetry strips from the emergency department showing development of Torsades

Diagnostic Testing

WBC	Hemoglobin	Platelets
9.9 k/mm^3	13 g/dL	200 k/mm^3

Na	K	Cl	CO_2	BUN	Cr	Glucose
138 mmol/L	4.1 mmol/L	102 mmol/L	30 mmol/L	12 mg/dL	0.9 mg/dL	154 mg/dL

Magnesium: 2.3 mg/dL
Acetaminophen, salicylates, and ethanol were undetectable

Ancillary Testing

CT head: negative for hemorrhage or masses

Hospital Course

The patient continued to have pause-dependent ventricular tachycardia. A temporary transvenous pacemaker was placed. In order to avoid diarrhea during the detoxification, the detoxification facility administered a cathartic shortly before starting the detoxification medication. The cathartic resulted in hypokalemia which proved somewhat difficult to treat. The dysrhythmias continued for several days, and ultimately resolved by hospital day 5. The QT normalized by hospital day 6.

Additional information was obtained regarding the detoxification regimen. The patient had received 4 doses of ibogaine (10.5 mg/kg per dose) and tabernanthe bark root extract (14 mg/kg per dose). The tabernanthe iboga root bark extract is comprised of 20–40% ibogaine, and 10–13% other alkaloids. Thus, he received a total of 750 mg of ibogaine and 1 g of the extract at the time he presented to the emergency department. The last dose of either xenobiotic was administered 3 h prior to presentation.

What Medications Can Induce Torsades and What Medications Can Be Used to Treat Torsades?

Almost any drug that induces QT prolongation can theoretically cause torsade de pointes. However, those who cause QT prolongation and tachycardia in overdose tend to have lower rates of torsades. The following table lists common drugs that can cause torsades.

Common causes of xenobiotic-induced torsades

Antiarrhythmics	Psychiatric drugs	Miscellaneous
Amiodarone	Amisulpride	Arsenic
Moricizine	Haloperidol	Astemizole
Procainamide	Chlorpromazine	Chloroquine
Quinidine	Citalopram	Cisapride
Sotalol	Perphenazine	Diphenhydramine
	Quetiapine	Erythromycin
	Thiothixene	Indapamide
	Thioridazine	Pentamidine
	Tricyclic antidepressants	Prochlorperazine
	Trifluoperazine	Terfenadine
	Ziprasidone	Thallium

Torsades de pointe is best treated with 2–4 g magnesium sulfate as an intravenous bolus. Overdrive pacing is another option.

What Is Ibogaine?

Ibogaine is a psychoactive indole alkaloid from the West African shrub *Tabernanthe iboga.* Traditionally, it was used in religious rituals by the Bwiti people in West Africa. It was known to western medicine for over a century and was initially marketed as a stimulant in France in the 1920s. However, in the 1960s, people began to experiment with its psychoactive properties and inadvertently discovered that heroin users did not display withdrawal symptoms after using ibogaine instead of heroin (Brown 2013).

What Is the Rationale for Using Ibogaine for Opioid Detoxification?

The discovery of ibogaine's anti-addictive properties is attributed to Howard Lotsof in 1962. Lotsof was a heroin user in New York City who organized and participated in a group who experimented with various psychoactive chemicals in order to find drugs with psychological benefits. Of the 20 individuals in Lotsof's group, seven were dependent on heroin; following their initial ingestion of ibogaine, 5 of those 7 reported that they entirely abstained from heroin use for at least 6 months thereafter. Lotsof himself noted that he did not suffer from heroin withdrawal or cravings while using ibogaine despite not using heroin for over 30 h (Brown 2013).

Animal studies show a decrease in morphine and cocaine self-administration following ibogaine and noribogaine (an active metabolite) administration (Glick and Maisonneuve 1998). Human data, however, is limited.

What Is the Typical Dose of Ibogaine and the Typical Ibogaine Detoxification Regimen?

Ibogaine is used most frequently as a single oral dose in the range of 10–25 mg/kg of body weight for the specific indication of detoxification from opioids. It is most commonly used in the form of the hydrochloride (HCl), which certificates of analysis typically indicate 95–98% pure (Alper et al. 2008). Ibogaine is also used in the form of alkaloid extracts or dried root bark. Lay providers administering ibogaine in nonmedical settings have accounted for the majority of treatments. In these cases, ibogaine is administered by nonmedical personnel who care for the patient in private settings (Alper et al. 2008). Most medical settings will conduct pretreatment EKGs and basic laboratory studies. In clinics in St Kitt's and Mexico, opioid-dependent patients are often converted to equivalent doses of orally administered short acting opioids. All centrally acting medications are tapered and discontinued for at least three serum half-lives prior to ibogaine initiation. Evaluation at these centers typically includes pretreatment Holter monitor and 12 lead EKG and continuous vital sign monitoring during treatment (Mash et al. 2000).

Is Ibogaine Legal in the United States?

Ibogaine is a schedule I substance in the United States, and similarly, is illegal in France, Denmark, Sweden, Belgium, Switzerland, and Australia. However, it is unregulated in most countries. US citizens may obtain Ibogaine abroad or over the internet. Recent case reports suggest that patients may be purchasing ibogaine over the internet and using it without the assistance of a healer or guide (O'Connell et al. 2015).

What Is the Proposed Mechanism of Action of Ibogaine?

The mechanism of action of ibogaine and its active metabolite noribogaine has not been fully elucidated. Ibogaine and noribogaine have distinct receptor profiles from each other. Both interact with NMDA, nicotinic (nACh), sigma, mu, and kappa opioid receptors. Ibogaine is a more potent NMDA receptor antagonist than noribogaine. Both act on opioid receptors, and it is hypothesized that changes in opioid receptor signaling may underlie its therapeutic effects. Despite ibogaine being more lipophilic than noribogaine, noribogaine seems to have greater effect on the *mu* receptor (Maciulaitis et al. 2008). However, recent data suggest that ibogaine and noribogaine may not be *mu* receptor agonists (Antonio et al. 2013). The exact receptor interaction and signaling pathway is still unknown. Ibogaine also causes release of presynaptic serotonin, prevents serotonin reuptake, and can act as a serotonin receptor agonist, which may mediate its hallucinogenic effects (Mash et al. 1998).

What Are Potential Toxicities Associated with Ibogaine?

Ingestion of ibogaine has been temporally related to several cases of sudden death. A systematic overview of all reported cases in the years between 1990 and 2008 found a total of 19 fatalities that occurred after ibogaine administration, mostly when administered for opioid detoxificationification or treatment of alcohol dependence. In 14 of these cases, post-mortem data demonstrated that the decedents suffered from preexisting medical conditions or were compromised by the additional intake of other drugs such as opioids and cocaine. The predominant autopsy findings involved the cardiovascular system and included: coronary artery sclerosis, hypertension, myocardial infarct, cardiac hypertrophy, and dilated cardiomyopathy. However, liver disease was also found in several cases including hepatitis, cirrhosis, and steatosis (Alper et al. 2012). This study spurred the development of pretreatment screening exams in the ibogaine community.

Common adverse effects are nausea, vomiting, and disturbing hallucinations. The most concerning effect is prolongation of the QT interval, potentially leading to fatal arrhythmias. Numerous case reports demonstrate QT prolongation with subsequent development of arrhythmias, including torsades de pointes (Vlaanderen et al. 2014; Paling et al. 2012; Pleskovic et al. 2012; Hoelen et al. 2009). In vitro studies demonstrate ibogaine may inhibit the hERG potassium channel in cardiac tissue, which may explain this phenomenon (Koenig and Hilber 2015; Alper et al. 2016; Thurner et al. 2014; Koenig et al. 2013).

Specialty-Specific Guidance

Emergency Medicine

- Torsades de pointes can occur with numerous medications, including ibogaine.
- Torsades de pointes is best treated with a bolus of intravenous magnesium

Addiction Medicine

- Ibogaine can cause blockade of the potassium channels, resulting in QT prolongation and increased risk of torsades.

Critical Care Medicine

- QT prolongation is one of the most common adverse reactions associated with ibogaine
- Emergency Medicine, Addiction Medicine, Cardiology, Critical Care

References

Alper KR, Lotsof HS, Kaplan CD. The ibogaine medical subculture. J Ethnopharmacol. 2008;115(1):9–24. Epub 2007.

Alper KR, Stajić M, Gill JR. Fatalities temporally associated with the ingestion of ibogaine. J Forensic Sci. 2012;57(2):398–412.

Alper K, Bai R, Liu N, Fowler SJ, Huang XP, Priori SG, Ruan Y. hERG blockade by Iboga alkaloids. Cardiovasc Toxicol. 2016;16(1):14–22.

Antonio T, Childers SR, Rothman RB, Dersch CM, King C, Kuehne M, Bornmann WG, Eshleman AJ, Janowsky A, Simon ER, Reith ME, Alper K. Effect of Iboga alkaloids on μ-opioid receptor-coupled G protein activation. PLoS One. 2013;8(10):e77262.

Brown TK. Ibogaine in the treatment of substance dependence. Curr Drug Abuse Rev. 2013;6(1):3–16.

Glick SD, Maisonneuve IS. Mechanisms of antiaddictive actions of ibogaine. Ann N Y Acad Sci. 1998;844:214–26.

Hoelen DW, Spiering W, Valk GD. Long-QT syndrome induced by the antiaddiction drug ibogaine. N Engl J Med. 2009;360(3):308–9.

Koenig X, Hilber K. The anti-addiction drug ibogaine and the heart: a delicate relation. Molecules. 2015;20(2):2208–28.

Koenig X, Kovar M, Rubi L, Mike AK, Lukacs P, Gawali VS, Todt H, Hilber K, Sandtner W. Anti-addiction drug ibogaine inhibits voltage-gated ionic currents: a study to assess the drug's cardiac ion channel profile. Toxicol Appl Pharmacol. 2013;273(2):259–68.

Maciulaitis R, Kontrimaviciute V, Bressolle FM, Briedis V. Ibogaine, an anti-addictive drug: pharmacology and time to go further in development. A narrative review. Hum Exp Toxicol. 2008;27(3):181–94.

Mash DC, Kovera CA, Buck BE, et al. Medication development of ibogaine as a pharmacotherapy for drug dependence. Ann N Y Acad Sci. 1998;844:274–92.

Mash DC, Kovera CA, Pablo J, Tyndale RF, Ervin FD, Williams IC, Singleton EG, Mayor M. Ibogaine: complex pharmacokinetics, concerns for safety, and preliminary efficacy measures. Ann N Y Acad Sci. 2000;914:394–401.

O'Connell CW, Gerona RR, Friesen MW, Ly BT. Internet-purchased ibogaine toxicity confirmed with serum, urine, and product content levels. Am J Emerg Med. 2015;33(7):985.e5–6.

Paling FP, Andrews LM, Valk GD, Blom HJ. Life-threatening complications of ibogaine: three case reports. Neth J Med. 2012;70(9):422–4.

Pleskovic A, Gorjup V, Brvar M, Kozelj G. Ibogaine-associated ventricular tachyarrhythmias. Clin Toxicol (Phila). 2012;50(2):157.

Thurner P, Stary-Weinzinger A, Gafar H, Gawali VS, Kudlacek O, Zezula J, Hilber K, Boehm S, Sandtner W, Koenig X. Mechanism of hERG channel block by the psychoactive indole alkaloid ibogaine. J Pharmacol Exp Ther. 2014;348(2):346–58.

Vlaanderen L, Martial LC, Franssen EJ, van der Voort PH, Oosterwerff E, Somsen GA. Cardiac arrest after ibogaine ingestion. Clin Toxicol (Phila). 2014;52(6):642–3.

Case 27
Hepatic Injury from a "Cultural Medicine"

1. What is on your list of differential diagnoses?
2. What is this "medication" and what is it used for?
3. What are side effects?
4. Is this substance associated with any type of withdrawal syndrome?
5. What is the treatment for intoxication with this substance?
6. What is cholestatic hepatitis?
7. What some of the other herbal supplements are associated with hepatotoxicity?
8. What type of hepatic injury occurs from pyrrolizidine alkaloids?
9. What are some other causes of drug-induced cholestasis?
10. How do anabolic steroids cause liver injury?

Abstract A 34-year-old female developed itching and jaundice after taking a "cultural medication" given to her by a friend. Laboratory studies from her initial emergency department evaluation suggest a cholestatic process. This chapter reviews herbal medications associated with hepatic injury and drugs that cause hepatic injury.

Keywords Cholestatic jaundice • Kratom • Anabolic steroids • Drug abuse • Opioids • Herbal medication

L.R. Dye et al. (eds.), *Case Studies in Medical Toxicology*,
DOI 10.1007/978-3-319-56449-4_27

History of Present Illness

A 34-year-old female presented to Hepatology clinic after being seen in the Emergency Department (ED) with pruritus and jaundice 2 weeks prior. She reported a history of chronic knee pain for which she had been taking a "cultural medication" given to her by a friend. She notes she began taking this medication 4–5 days prior to presenting to the ED and first developed itching and then noted some yellowing of her skin. She denied abdominal pain, vomiting, fevers, chills, or myalgias.

Past Medical History	Chronic knee pain No history of liver disease
Medications	"Cultural medication" given to her by friend for pain is the only medication she has been taking, but stopped taking this after evaluation in ED She reports no use of prescription medications, over-the-counter medications, or herbal supplements
Allergies	NKDA
Social History	Denies tobacco use Denies alcohol use Denies recreational drug use
Family History	No family history of liver disease

Physical Examination

Blood pressure	Heart rate	Respiratory rate	Temperature	O_2 saturation
130/50 mmHg	85 bpm	15 breaths/min	37 °C (98.6 °F)	97% (room air)

General: Alert, sitting on stretcher in no acute distress. WDWN. Appears stated age and well-groomed.

HEENT: Mild sclera icterus; pupils equal, round, and reactive to light. No nystagmus and extraocular movements intact on direct testing.

Cardiovascular: Normal rate; no murmurs, gallops, or rubs. 2+ pulses in all four extremities.

Pulmonary: Clear to auscultation bilaterally with no wheezes, rales, rhonchi. No tachypnea, stridor, accessory muscle use.

Abdomen: Non-tender, normal active bowel sounds. No distension or fluid wave. No hepatosplenomegaly appreciated.

Skin: Mild jaundice, warm and dry. No rashes or lesions noted.

Neurologic: Awake and alert. Oriented x4. No asterixis. Normal muscular tone. Cranial nerves 2–12 intact on direct testing. Strength 5/5 all four extremities and symmetric sensation to light touch throughout.

Diagnostic Testing

Emergency Department Visit

AST: 40 IU/L
ALT: 73 IU/L
Alkaline phosphatase: 173 IU/L
Total bilirubin: 13.4 mg/dL
CBC and BMP: "normal"

Office Visit

AST: 36 IU/L
ALT: 74 IU/L
T bilirubin: 11 mg/dL

WBC	Hemoglobin	Hematocrit	Platelets	Differential
9.5 k/mm^3	12 g/dL		215 k/mm^3	

Na	K	Cl	CO_2	BUN/Cr
139 mmol/L	4.2 mmol/L	102 mmol/L	24 mmol/L	8/0.9 mg/dL

Ancillary Testing

Abdominal US: normal
Magnetic Resonance Cholangiopancreatography (MRCP): negative
Liver biopsy: demonstrated eosinophilic infiltrates
Hepatitis serology: negative
Autoimmune hepatitis evaluation: negative

What Is on Your List of Differential Diagnoses?

- Cholestatic process
- Hepatic necrosis
- Falsely elevated bilirubin secondary to metabolite of naproxyn that cross reacts with total bilirubin testing
- Anabolic steroid use

What Is Kratom and What Is It Used for?

- Kratom (*Mitragynia speciosa*) is a tree found in Southeast Asia.
- Fresh leaves from the tree are often chewed or brewed into a tea. Dried leaves can be ground into a powder or used whole for teas, as well as smoked.
- Kratom has both stimulant and opioid effects (Shellard 1989)
- Onset of action is approximately 5–10 min after leaf chewing and effects last from 2–5 h.
- Kratom is taken for pain control and is used as a treatment for opioid withdrawal (Boyer et al. 2008; Prozialeck et al. 2012; Suwanlert 1975)
- Kratom contains multiple active alkaloids. Mitragynine and 7-hydroxymitragynine are the primary active agents that act on opioid (μ and κ) receptors (Prozialeck et al. 2012).
- A lower level of 7-hydroxymitragynine compared to mitragynin is found in kratom, but 7-hydroxymitragynine is 46 fold more potent than mitragynin (Matsumoto et al. 2004; Prozialeck et al. 2012).
- "Krypton" is a kratom-based product with added o-desmethyltramadol and is marketed as a more potent form of kratom (Arndt et al. 2011). Some reports indicate there is also a product marketed as "Krypton" that is a combination of caffeine and O-desmethyltramadol (Reys 2013).

What Are Side Effects of Kratom Use?

- Suwanlert reviewed symptoms noted with chronic kratom users in Thailand in the 1970s (1975). In this population, kratom was used to enhance productivity in manual laborers. Users either chewed the leaf directly or made tea. Side effects noted by the author and users included dry mouth, frequent urination, constipation, darkening of the skin (specifically the cheeks), anorexia, insomnia, and weight loss. Some patients were noted to develop psychosis, as well. It is unclear if the kratom use unmasked underlying psychosis or directly caused the psychosis (Suwanlert 1975).
- A few case reports of seizures following kratom use have been published; however, most of these cases involve an additional xenobiotic, so it is difficult to know if the causative agent was kratom, another substance, or a combination of drug effects (Boyer et al. 2008; Nelsen et al. 2010).
- There is an isolated case report suggesting a possible association between the onset of primary hypothyroidism and kratom use; however, this is a loose association from the data presented and warrants further investigation (Sheleg and Collins 2011)
- Intrahepatic cholestasis was reported by Kapp et al. (2011) in a case where an otherwise healthy 25-year-old male used kratom for 2 weeks, discontinued use, and subsequently developed jaundice and pruritus. Much like this case, symptoms and laboratory abnormalities improved over time (Kapp et al. 2011).

- One report by Neerman et al. (2013) describes a possible kratom-related death in a patient who reportedly consumed liquid kratom the night before he was found dead. The patient was known to have chronic pain and an opioid abuse history, for which he took kratom. Elevated levels of mitragynine (0.60 mg/L) were noted in post-mortem whole blood and autopsy findings were similar to those noted in opioid-related deaths. Other medications noted on post-mortem whole blood testing included: dextromethorphan, diphenhydramine, temazepam, and 7-amino-clonazepam.
- Another report details the death of a 24 year-old who was noted to have mitragynine on GC-MS testing of peripheral blood, central blood, in the liver, vitreous fluid and urine. Additionally, venlafaxine, diphenhydramine, and mirtazapine were also detected in the patient's system (McIntyre et al. 2015).
- There is little evidence in the literature detailing mitragynine blood concentrations and clinical effects.

Is Kratom Associated with Any Type of Withdrawal Syndrome?

- Chronic users of kratom report symptoms of withdrawal with abstinence.
- These symptoms mimic opioid withdrawal in nature and involve nausea, abdominal cramping, diarrhea, and diaphoresis (Boyer et al. 2008; Galbis-Reig 2016; Sheleg and Collins 2011).

What Is the Treatment for Kratom Intoxication?

- The treatment for kratom intoxication should be largely supportive.
- Patients with severe sympathomimetic symptoms can be treated with benzodiazepines with close monitoring for respiratory depression given the synergistic activities in conjunction with opioid agonism.
- There is inconsistent data regarding the effectiveness of naloxone in reversing the opioid effects of kratom. However, naloxone should be considered in patients with insufficient respirations. If naloxone is ineffective, mechanical support may be necessary (Rosenbaum et al. 2012).
- Of note, kratom has been reported to cause serious respiratory depression in case series when mixed with other substances such as tramadol. In these cases, the opioid agonism effect is much larger and has resulted in several deaths (Kronstrand et al. 2011).

What Is Cholestatic Hepatitis?

- Cholestatic hepatitis is the toxin-induced impairment of bile synthesis and flow.
  - This occurs from direct toxin damage to canalicular cells, but doesn't always affect hepatocytes (AST and ALT may be normal).
  - Alkaline phosphatase and bilirubin levels are elevated
- Symptoms and clinical findings often include dark urine, pruritus, and jaundice
- There is often a period of 2–24 weeks between initial exposure and onset of symptoms.

What some of the Other Herbal Supplements Are Associated with Hepatotoxicity?

- Pennyroyal oil (*Hedeoma pulegioides*; *Mentha pulegium*)
- Chaparral (*Larrea tridentate*)
- Germander (*Teucrium chamaedrys*)
- Kava kava (*Piper methysticum*)
- Pyrrolizidine alkaloids
  - Borage aka: *Borago officinalis*
  - Comfrey aka: *Symphytum officinale*

What Type of Hepatic Injury Occurs from Pyrrolizidine Alkaloids?

- Veno-occlusive disease results from intimal thickening of the terminal hepatic venules from toxin-induced injury to the endothelium. This results in edema and nonthrombotic obstruction (Ridker 1989).
- Fibrosis can develop in the central and sublobular veins.
- Sinusoidal dilation in the centrilobular areas is associated with hepatic necrosis and cellular injury.

What are some Other Causes of Drug-Induced Cholestasis?

- Anabolic steroids
- Estrogen
- 4,4′-methylenedianiline
- Rapeseed oil aniline
- Cyclosporine

How Do Anabolic Steroids Cause Liver Injury?

- Anabolic steroids have been associated with two types of liver injury, peliosis hepatitis and hepatocellular adenoma and adenocarcinomas.
- Peliosis hepatitis is a form of liver injury where blood-filled cysts fill the liver without inflammatory changes; sinusoidal congestion can also occur.
- Diagnosis of peliosis hepatitis is difficult to make antemortem. The diagnosis should be considered in patients with signs of hepatomegaly and liver function abnormalities in the setting of anabolic steroid use (McDonald and Speicher 1978).
- Peliosis hepatitis may be reversible with cessation of anabolic steroid use (McDonald and Speicher 1978).
- Liver adenomas and adenocarcinomas may develop in patients with anabolic steroid use (Socas et al. 2005).
- Though controversial, it is thought that non-malignant hepatic adenomas have potential to become malignant adenocarcinomas (Socas et al. 2005).
- Very large non-malignant adenomas have potential to cause serious illness or death from bleeding, liver failure, or rupture.

Case Conclusion

In this case, the patient took a friend's "cultural medication," kratom (*Mitragynia speciosa),* for chronic knee pain. She developed choelstatic jaundice shortly after starting this therapy and the symptoms resolved spontaneously with discontinuation of the "cultural medication"/herbal supplement. The use and side effects of kratom were discussed, as well as other causes of cholestatsis and herbal supplement-related hepatic injury.

Specialty-Specific Guidance

Internal Medicine/Family Medicine

- Ask patients with chronic pain about the use of herbal supplements or alternative medications.
- Cholestatic jaundice is frequently associated with plant alkaloids and anabolic steroid use.
- If patients develop symptoms of cholestatic jaundice or hepatitis, stop all potential hepatotoxic agents, including herbal supplements and alternative medicines.
- Refer to gastroenterology for further evaluation.

Emergency Medicine

- A detailed social and medication history needs to be taken. This should include obtaining information about use of over-the-counter medications, herbal supplements, and alternative medicine therapies.
- The clinical presentation of acute/chronic kratom use varies widely from stimulatory to opioid-like effect.
- Consider the use of other hepatotoxic agents and infectious causes of liver injury.
- Close follow-up with gastroenterology should be arranged if discharging any patient with acute hepatitis. If unable to arrange follow-up, consider admission for observation.

Toxicology

- Obtain detailed occupational/environmental, social, and medication history. Be certain to include questions regarding the use of herbal/dietary supplements and alternative medicine therapies.
- Consider polypharmacy as the cause of liver injury, as multiple agents can cause hepatotoxicity.
- Potentially serious toxicity is rare and has been reported at doses greater than 15 grams, but in these cases, co-ingestants were present and the clinical effects were most likely caused by the co-ingestants.
- Use of kratom in high doses (>15 gm) chronically is associated with the development cholestatic jaundice.
- "Krypton" is a kratom-based product with the addition of exogenous o-desmethyltramadol and is marketed as a more potent form of kratom.
- Kratom has been associated with new onset seizures and the development of primary hypothyroidism in published case reports. This is something to be aware of when evaluating patients who have new onset seizures or hypothyroidism and use kratom.

References

Arndt T, Claussen U, Gussregen B, Schrofel S, Sturzer B, Werle A, et al. Kratom alkaloids and O-desmethyltramadol in urine of a "Krypton" herbal mixture consumer. Forensic Sci Int. 2011;208(1–3):47–52.

Boyer E, Babu K, Adkins J, McCurdy C, Halpern J. Self-treatment of opioid withdrawal using kratom (Mitragynia speciosa korth). Addiction. 2008;103(6):1048–50.

Galbis-Reig D. A case report of kratom addiction and withdrawal. WMJ. 2016;115(1):49–52.

Kapp F, Maurer H, Auwarter V, Winkelmann M, Hermanns-Clausen M. Intrahepatic cholestasis following abuse of powdered kratom (Mitragynina speciosa). J Med Toxicol. 2011;7(3):227–31.

Kronstrand R, Roman M, Thelander G, Eriksson A. Unintentional fatal intoxications with mitragynine and O-desmethyl- tramadol from the herbal blend Krypton. J Anal Toxicol. 2011;35(4):242–7.

Matsumoto K, Horie S, Ishikawa H, Takayama H, Aimi N, Ponglux D, et al. Antinociceptive effect of 7-hydroxymitragynine in mice: discovery of an orally active opioid analgesic from the Thai medicinal herb Mitragyna speciosa. Life Sci. 2004;74(14):2143–55.

McDonald EC, Speicher CE. Peliosis hepatis associated with administration of oxymetholone. JAMA. 1978;240(3):243–4.

McIntyre IM, Trochta A, Stolberg S, Campman SC. Mitragynine "Kratom" related fatality: a case report with postmortem concentrations. J Anal Toxicol. 2015;39(2):152–5.

Neerman M, Frost R, Deking J. A drug fatality involving kratom. J Forensic Sci. 2013;58(s1):S278–9.

Nelsen J, Lapoint J, Hodgman M, Aldous K. Seizure and coma following kratom (Mitragynina speciosa korth) exposure. J Med Toxicol. 2010;6:424–6.

Prozialeck WC, Jivan JK, Andurkar SV. Pharmacology of kratom: an emerging botanical agent with stimulant, analgesic and opioid-like effects. J Am Osteopath Assoc. 2012;112(12):792–9.

Reys L. Krypton Kratom Review—DO NOT buy these pills. 2013. http://kratomonline.org/krypton-kratom-review/. Accessed 3 Oct 2015.

Ridker P, McDermott W. Comfrey herb tea and hepatic veno-occlusive disease. Lancet. 1989;1(8639):657–8.

Rosenbaum CD, Carreiro SP, Babu KM. Here today, gone tomorrow … and back again? A review of herbal marijuana alternatives (K2, Spice), synthetic cathinones (bath salts), kratom, Salvia divinorum, methoxetamine, and piperazines. J Med Toxicol. 2012;8(1):15–32. doi:10.1007/s13181-011-0202-2.

Sheleg S, Collins G. A coincidence of addiction to "kratom" and severe primary hypothyroidism. J Addict Med. 2011;5(4):300–1.

Shellard E. Ethanopharmacology of Kratom and the Mitragyna alkaloids. J Ethnopharmacol. 1989;25:123–4.

Socas L, Zumbado M, Perez-Luzardo O, Ramos A, et al. Hepatocellular adenomas associated with anabolic androgenic steroid abuse in bodybuilders: a report of two cases and a review of the literature. Br J Sports Med. 2005;39(5):e27.

Suwanlert S. A study of kratom eaters in Thailand. Bull Narc. 1975;27(3):21–7.

Case 28
Glyphosate Toxicity

1. What is glyphosate, and where is it found?
2. What is the effect of concentration on the severity of symptoms?
3. How does glyphosate toxicity occur?
4. What are the clinical manifestations of glyphosate toxicity?
5. What treatment options exist for glyphosate poisoning?

Abstract Glyphosate is an herbicide used by both amateurs and professionals. It is commonly co-formulated with a surfactant. Ingestions of glyphosate can result in significant gastrointestinal hemorrhage due to its corrosive injury. Metabolic acidosis and noncardiogenic pulmonary edema, along with renal and hepatic impairment, can occur. This case describes a male who ingested a concentrated glyphosate product.

Keywords Glyphosate • Metabolic acidosis • Renal failure • GI bleed

History of Present Illness

A 50-year-old male with a history of bipolar disorder, who recently moved to the US from Taiwan, presented approximately 12 h after an intentional ingestion of 6.5 ounces of 50.2% glyphosate with isopropylamine salt. He developed nausea and vomiting and sought medical care. In the emergency department, he was noted to be tachycardic and tachypneic. He received IV fluids and fomepizole for a metabolic acidosis and was transferred to a tertiary care medical center.

L.R. Dye et al. (eds.), *Case Studies in Medical Toxicology*,
DOI 10.1007/978-3-319-56449-4_28

Past Medical History	Bipolar disorder
Medications	Lithium
Allergies	Non-known medication allergies
Family History	Unable to be obtained
Social History	Current smoker. No history of ethanol use or illicit drug use

Physical Examination

Blood pressure	**Heart rate**	**Respiratory rate**	**Temperature**	**O_2 saturation**
150/80 mmHg	120 bpm	34 breaths/min	36.4 °C (97.6°F)	94% on 3 L/min

General: Well-developed, well-nourished, well-hydrated ill-appearing male in moderate acute distress

HEENT: The conjunctivae are pink, and the sclaera are anicteric. Pupils are 3 mm and reactive bilaterally. There are moist mucosal membranes

Cardiovascular: tachycardic with a regular rhythm. No murmurs

Pulmonary: coarse lung sounds bilaterally. Tachypnea.

Abdomen: soft with epigastric tenderness. No rebound or guarding. Bowel sounds are normal

Neurologic: somnolent. Moans to painful stimuli. He moves all extremities spontaneously, but does not follow commands

Skin: warm, diaphoretic, and well-perfused.

What Is Glyphosate, and Where Is It Found?

Glyphosate is a phosphorous-containing pesticide that is available in various concentrations and is one of the most common products used in agriculture today. It is applied to the majority of corn and soy crops grown in the United States and is commonly used as a household herbicide. Interestingly, it is one of the first herbicides against which crops have been genetically modified in order to increase their tolerance. It has recently gained media attention when the International Agency for Research on Cancer (IARC) gave it a 2A designation, as "probably carcinogenic to humans." This is a subject of ongoing debate for food safety, as other independent expert panels disagree with the IARC assessment (Williams et al. 2016).

What Is the Effect of Concentration on the Severity of Symptoms?

Glyphosate herbicides are formulated in a wide variety of concentrations, ranging from 1% ready-to-use sprays to 50% super concentrate. Even high concentrations are available for household use and are intended for dilution prior to application. The more concentrated the solution, the more severe the symptoms are likely to be. Ingestions of 30 mL of 41% glyphosate solutions have produced nausea, vomiting, diarrhea, and a burning sensation in the throat, but generally do not cause severe symptoms. Ingestions of more concentrated solutions or larger volumes are more likely to cause serious toxicity (Bradberry et al. 2004).

Case Continued

In the emergency department, he received 8 mg of ondansetron and 2 L of normal saline. An electrocardiogram revealed intraventricular conduction delay prompting the administration of 150 mEq of sodium bicarbonate. Fomepizole was ordered, but not given prior to transfer.

Upon arrival in the ICU, the patient was emergently intubated. He was noted to be anuric with evidence of shock, requiring norepinephrine and vasopressin infusions. He was anuric and hypernatremic and was started on continuous renal replacement therapy.

How Does Glyphosate Toxicity Occur?

The mechanism by which glyphosate causes poisoning is unclear, as is the relative contribution of glyphosate itself versus its varied surfactant vehicles (Bradberry et al. 2004; Vincent and Davidson 2015). Available surfactants include polyoxyethyleneamine (POEA), polyethoxylated alkyletheramine, polyoxyphosphate amine, trimethylethoxypolyoxypropyl ammonium chloride, and ethoxylated phosphate ester. Most evidence suggests the surfactant, rather than glyphosate itself, is the toxin (Bradberry et al. 2004).

What Are the Clinical Manifestations of Glyphosate Toxicity?

Severe glyphosate ingestions can result in GI symptoms (nausea, vomiting diarrhea) and odynophagia. Corrosive effects can be seen, including ulcerations, necrosis, and gastrointestinal hemorrhage with shock (Bates and Edwards 2013; Talbot et al.

1991; Chen et al. 2013). Noncardiogenic pulmonary edema, pneumomediastinum, and subcutaneous emphysema have been described following aspiration of glyphosate-containing products. Renal and hepatic failure, along with central nervous system depression and metabolic acidosis, can be observed (Talbot et al. 1991; Tominack et al. 1991).

Case Continued

A computerized tomography (CT) scan of the head was negative for acute pathology, and a CT scan of the abdomen and pelvis revealed circumferential gas along the small bowel lumen throughout the upper quadrants, possibly representing pneumatosis intestinalis. No free air was identified, although there was a diffuse ileus without definitive bowel obstruction. Dense consolidation was noted in the right lung base.

Blood cultures obtained on admission grew gram negative bacilli. On the first hospital day, the vasopressors were weaned, but the patient continued to have a distended abdomen. In light of the CT findings and increasing lactic acid, the patient was taken to the operating room for a diagnostic laparoscopy. The bowel appeared normal.

Over the next several days, the patient remained anuric and comatose. Thrombocytopenia developed. On the fourth hospital day, the patient developed a GI bleed requiring transfusion of packed red blood cells and platelets. Endoscopy revealed patchy hemorrhagic exudative appearance of the gastric body with a large amount of blood in the stomach.

On hospital day six, the patient underwent an exploratory laparotomy with abdominal wash out. An area of ischemic bowel was identified and was resected. The patient was taken back to the operating room the following day where laparotomy revealed a diffusely ischemic distal ileum and cecum and underwent a small bowel resection with right hemicolectomy. On hospital day 9, the patient underwent tracheostomy and an ileostomy with closure of the abdominal wall.

On hospital day 19, the patient underwent repeat CT scan of the abdomen and pelvis, which revealed significant hemoperitoneum.

Repeat endoscopy on hospital day 26 revealed a normal esophagus without obvious etiology of GI bleed. An ileoscopy through the stoma revealed large clot with old blood without any clear source of the bleeding. The stoma was without evidence of bleeding.

What Treatment Options Exist for Glyphosate Poisoning?

There are no specific treatment options, other than aggressive supportive care including fluid resuscitation and correction of metabolic abnormalities. Gastrointestinal decontamination is not advised due to the risk of worsening corrosive injury. No antidote exists. Lipid emulsion therapy has been suggested, but convincing data supporting any beneficial effect from lipid at this point are lacking. Some reports suggest benefit from extracorporeal removal.

Case Conclusion

The patient continued to have GI bleeding requiring multiple transfusions and underwent mesenteric angiogram, which did not reveal any clear etiology of bleeding. Because it was felt that further transfusions were futile and surgery was not an option to stop further bleeding, the family ultimately decided to withdraw care and the patient expired shortly thereafter.

Specialty-Specific Guidance

Critical Care Medicine

- Glyphosate is a commonly available herbicide which, if ingested in large quantities or high concentrations, causes corrosive injury and multisystem organ failure.
- Treatment is supportive. No antidotal therapy has been proven to be beneficial, although hemodialysis may confer some benefit.

Emergency Medicine

- Glyphosate is a very common household herbicide, and available concentrations vary widely.
- Large volume or high concentration ingestions may have a poor outcome.
- Gastrointestinal decontamination may worsen corrosive injury.

References

Bates N, Edwards N. Glyphosate toxicity in animals. Clin Toxicol. 2013;51:1243.
Bradberry SM, Proudfoot AT, Vale JA. Glyphosate poisoning. Toxicol Rev. 2004;23:159–67.
Chen HH, Lin JL, Huang WH. Spectrum of corrosive esophageal injury after intentional paraquat or glyphosate-surfactant herbicide ingestion. Int J Gen Med. 2013;14:677–83.
Garlich FM, Goldman M, Pepe J, et al. Hemodialysis clearance of glyphosate following a life-threatening ingestion of glyphosate-surfactant herbicide. Clin Toxicol. 2014;52:66–71.

Gil HW, Park JS, Park SH, et al. Effect of intravenous lipid emulsion in patients with acute glyphosate intoxication. Clin Toxicol. 2013;51:767–71.

Talbot AR, Shiaw MH, Huang JS, et al. Acute poisoning with a glyphosate-surfactant herbicide ('Roundup'): a review of 93 cases. Hum Exp Toxicol. 1991;19:1–8.

Thakur DS, Khot R, Joshi PP, et al. Glyphosate poisoning with acute pulmonary edema. Toxicol Int. 2014;21:328–30.

Tominack RL, Yang GY, Tsai WJ, et al. Taiwan National Poison Center survey of glyphosate-surfactant herbicide ingestions. J Toxicol Clin Toxicol. 1991;29:91–109.

Vincent K, Davidson C. The toxicity of glyphosate alone and glyphosate-surfactant mixtures to western toad (Anaxyrus boreas) tadpoles. Environ Toxicol Chem. 2015;34:2791–5.

Williams GM, Aardema M, Acquavella J. A review of the carcinogenic potential of glyphosate by four independent expert panels and comparison to the IARC assessment. Crit Rev Toxicol. 2016;46:3–20.

Index

L.R. Dye et al. (eds.), *Case Studies in Medical Toxicology*,
DOI 10.1007/978-3-319-56449-4

CPSIA information can be obtained
at www.ICGtesting.com
Printed in the USA
LVOW05*0141110118
562565LV00001B/72/P

9 783319 564470